M000239118

Developing Identity, Strengths, and Self-Perception for Young Adults with Autism Spectrum Disorder

other books in the series

Independence, Social, and Study Strategies for Young Adults with Autism Spectrum Disorder
The BASICS College Curriculum
Michelle Rigler, Amy Rutherford and Emily Quinn
ISBN 978 1 84905 787 5
eISBN 978 1 78450 060 3

of related interest

A Freshman Survival Guide for College Students with Autism Spectrum Disorders
The Stuff Nobody Tells You About!
Haley Moss
Foreword by Susan J. Moreno
ISBN 978 1 84905 984 8
eISBN 978 0 85700 922 7

Top Tips for Asperger Students
How to Get the Most Out of University and College
Rosemary Martin
ISBN 978 1 84905 140 8
eISBN 978 0 85700 341 6

Succeeding as a Student in the STEM Fields with an Invisible Disability
A College Handbook for Science, Technology, Engineering, and Math Students with Autism, ADD, Affective Disorders, or Learning Difficulties and their Families
Christy Oslund
ISBN 978 1 84905 947 3
eISBN 978 0 85700 817 6

Helping Students with Autism Spectrum Disorder Express their Thoughts and Knowledge in Writing
Tips and Exercises for Developing Writing Skills
Elise Geither and Lisa Meeks
ISBN 978 1 84905 996 1
eISBN 978 0 85700 980 7

Supporting College and University Students with Invisible Disabilities
A Guide for Faculty and Staff Working with Students with Autism, AD/HD, Language Processing Disorders, Anxiety, and Mental Illness
Christy Oslund
ISBN 978 1 84905 955 8
eISBN 978 0 85700 785 8

Developing Identity, Strengths, and Self-Perception for Young Adults with Autism Spectrum Disorder

The BASICS College Curriculum

MICHELLE RIGLER,
AMY RUTHERFORD,
and EMILY QUINN

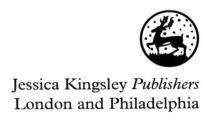

Jessica Kingsley *Publishers*
London and Philadelphia

First published in 2015
by Jessica Kingsley Publishers
73 Collier Street
London N1 9BE, UK
and
400 Market Street, Suite 400
Philadelphia, PA 19106, USA

www.jkp.com

Copyright © Michelle Rigler, Amy Rutherford and Emily Quinn 2015

Front cover image source: iStockphoto®.

All rights reserved. No part of this publication may be reproduced in any material form (including photocopying of any pages other than those marked with a ⬇, storing it in any medium by electronic means and whether or not transiently or incidentally to some other use of this publication) without the written permission of the copyright owner except in accordance with the provisions of the Copyright, Designs and Patents Act 1988 or under the terms of a licence issued by the Copyright Licensing Agency Ltd, Saffron House, 6–10 Kirby Street, London EC1N 8TS. Applications for the copyright owner's written permission to reproduce any part of this publication should be addressed to the publisher.

All pages marked ⬇ can be downloaded at www.jkp.com/catalogue/book/9781849057974 for personal use with this program, but may not be reproduced for any other purposes without the permission of the publisher.

Warning: The doing of an unauthorised act in relation to a copyright work may result in both a civil claim for damages and criminal prosecution.

Library of Congress Cataloging in Publication Data
A CIP catalog record for this book is available from the Library of Congress

British Library Cataloguing in Publication Data
A CIP catalogue record for this book is available from the British Library

ISBN 978 1 84905 797 4
eISBN 978 1 78450 095 5

Printed and bound in Great Britain

CONTENTS

ACKNOWLEDGEMENTS

EMILY QUINN

To my partner, and all my friends and family—I wish to express an infinite thank you for your support and love. It is because of all of you that I have been able to follow through with The BASICS College Curriculum, and I could not be more grateful to you for that.

Michelle and Amy, thank you for making me laugh every day and lending your brilliant insight to this project. I am constantly humbled by your knowledge and work ethic.

And to Rebecca—you have made us so proud. Thank you for your effort to pursue, achieve, and maintain such strong, independent, and wise self-identity, as it has helped guide us throughout the course of developing this curriculum. I cannot wait to see what the future holds for you.

MICHELLE RIGLER

To my parents who are always my biggest cheerleaders, thank you for cheering so loud my whole life, and to my husband, Chad, and my beautiful and brilliant children—Dylan, Cameron and Sydney— thank you for making me want to be a better person every day that I wake up. Because you all support and encourage me so much, I have been able to see this project through.

Amy and Emily, I am consistently in awe by your intelligence, compassion, and commitment to our work. The lives of young adults with ASD will be greatly impacted by your work and your passion and your ability to just "get it."

Finally to Cody—with every interaction I have with you, I learn more and more. Your brief comment in the middle of our conversation three years ago in which you said "I am everything polar negative about autism" created a visceral reaction in me. That single comment was the impetus for creating the entire second book in this series. You have grown into such a strong, confident, genuine, and gentle young man. I cannot thank you enough for lending me your knowledge on this incredibly important project.

AMY RUTHERFORD

To my mom and dad, thank you for always encouraging me to be all that I can be. To Zach, thank you for supporting my wild ideas, late-night work sessions and making sure I take the time to laugh every day. To all my family and friends, the constant love and support has shaped my life in more ways than you can imagine, and I am grateful for each and every one of you.

A special thanks to the many students who have come through my office: I cannot wait to see what the future holds for each and every one of you as you begin to recognize the amazing potential each one of you holds. The stories you share of your personal growth through this curriculum has made such an impact on the work we do.

To the staff and volunteers at the Chattanooga Autism Center, thank you for the work you put into serving the autism community. To Michelle, thank you for seeing something in me so many years ago. You have been instrumental to who I am as a professional, and helped to spark my passion for autism. To Emily, without you this project would never have been completed. Thank you for keeping us grounded and focused throughout this venture!

INTRODUCTION

As young adults with Autism Spectrum Disorder (ASD) hear of and learn about this particular diagnosis, they tend to respond to the diagnosis based on how they see others react. It is responsible to recognize the period of time following the notification of the diagnosis as a time when parents and caregivers may feel afraid, frustrated, or even grief. However, maintaining this view could foster feelings of shame in the individual with the diagnosis. By shifting focus to identify the strengths and positive impact of ASD within each individual, a person with ASD may truly embrace the diagnosis and become a strong self-advocate during the influential identity development stage that many young adults experience during college years.

This installment of the BASICS College Curriculum is designed to help people with ASD reframe their self-perception of their diagnosis. While there are some significant challenges associated with having the diagnosis of ASD, too often the truly positive qualities represented by individuals on the spectrum are overlooked. Knowing this, readers are encouraged to reflect on the personal stories they have been told, either through the words or actions of others, throughout key times in their lives. Through an academic-based approach, students make connections about shared experiences and have the opportunity to reflect on their experiences and replace the negative thoughts with positive thoughts about their own personal qualities.

Research has shown that people with ASD have many positive qualities that can contribute greatly to groups. Some of these qualities include systemized thinking, dependability, honesty, and detailed thinking, to name a few. These qualities are often overshadowed by the difficulties in the social arena. If readers spend as much time examining their strengths as they do hearing about their weaknesses, it is the hope that they will in turn develop a more positive self-perception. People throughout history that have been called geniuses have carried many of the same qualities that would be considered autistic by today's standards. Some of our greatest thinkers (see Chapter 4) have been highly creative and detailed but took a different path to arrive at conclusions, often coming up with solutions to problems that others could not see. This message is carried throughout this guide to help readers recognize and embrace the truly beneficial qualities inherent in ASD.

Throughout the first half of this guide, students spend time reflecting on the negative diagnostic language, media reflections, self-talk, etc. and working to reframe that negative language to recognize and own the positive qualities of ASD. Visual and hands-on work allows participants to challenge their self-perceptions while engaging with academic and literature-based evidence of the positive qualities of ASD. Students are encouraged to identify the strengths they recognize within themselves in order for them to then commit to changing their negative self-perceptions. Chapter 1 introduces the notion of personal stories and how they have been developed through life experiences. Participants are challenged to reflect on past stories and use new confidence to control the rewriting of their own personal story. Chapter 2 follows the discussion of personal stories by addressing the negative aspect of diagnostic language. Readers are encouraged to view the diagnostic language through a different lens that focuses on identity through strength-based language. Chapter 3 begins the study of what society is told about ASD through the various methods of the media. After examining what society is told through newspapers, television, journals, social media, etc., readers are invited to begin educating others about ASD and the positive impact on their own lives. In Chapter 4, the researched and proven strengths of individuals with ASD are outlined and discussed thoroughly. Participants will be urged to identify the strengths they see in themselves and others with ASD leading to the reframing of the view of ASD.

To begin the second half of this curriculum, readers are challenged to recognize the topic areas or social situations that make them feel calm, content, or anxious. This allows them to develop a self-monitoring system in order to be more in control of their own emotions and behavior. Recognizing their strengths and potential pitfalls, as well as identifying characteristics that work to define them is imperative as readers begin developing a core identity model. This model prompts students to focus on the aspects of their identity and their values that truly define who they are as a person. The elements that guide how students think about situations and make decisions, how they perceive themselves or others, and their behaviors or reactions to others will guide the discussions and work. These features will be challenged and discussed in an effort to identify the core elements of their identity. Once these are outlined, participants will be challenged to re-examine their black-and-white belief system that is often inherent in people with ASD. Finally, after developing, challenging, and finalizing the core identity features, readers will work to see the gray hues between the black and white of every belief and situation.

Reflecting on the positive view from interactions throughout their lives, students are challenged further to identify their personality strengths and how those strengths can contribute to success. Understanding their personality is the first step in beginning to see strengths within groups when working with others both in the classroom and in a job. By recognizing their personality characteristics and the potential benefit involved in a group or work setting, readers will learn to identify the personality qualities of others to allow them to build solid work groups. Chapter 5 begins this work with identifying and understanding various personality types. Recognizing the positive impact of all types of personalities will be addressed as a key component in building good partnerships in college, work, teams, or social groups. Chapter 6 then focuses heavily on identifying the features of personality that readers are committed to adhering to regardless of outside pressures. While it is imperative to hold true to these features, it is also important to recognize the potential detrimental effects of holding too tightly to these features without regard to relationships. Chapter 7 addresses the hidden social rules that are often a source of confusion for people with ASD. These rules are introduced and the purpose behind them discussed to help readers make sense of the social tools needed for success. Finally, in Chapter 8, the authors help to ease the process of transitioning to the next phase in the BASICS College Curriculum with an emphasis on employment as participants are introduced to the Career Continuum. This continuum introduces the notion that a career is a process with multiple steps and contacts. In discussions regarding the Career Continuum, readers are encouraged to consider community service, job shadowing, mentoring, internships, and mock interviews to lead up to the career of choice. Readers are introduced to the idea of a Career Continuum that outlines all the needed steps to take to move towards a successful career. Readers will examine the benefits of community service, job shadowing, mentors, and job search skills.

This guide will present a set of tools throughout each chapter to help students with ASD fill their "social toolbox." The impact of ASD is highly individualized, so throughout this text, various methods will be used to convey the important messages. As with any curriculum, the tools can be offered, but it is essentially up to the reader to choose to use them properly. Our primary method of reinforcing these concepts for the purposes of this guide will be to remind the students that in any situation and in any endeavor, it is always important to remember the BASICS.

The BASICS chart will be the conclusion to each chapter (see Table I.1 on page 13). Readers will have a visual representation of the subject matter that is to be reflected upon in the same pattern for each chapter. While primarily providing a reflection on the understanding of the subject, the BASICS chart offers an opportunity for readers to perform a confidential self-evaluation. Following the self-evaluation, readers should be prepared to develop a set of short-term goals based on the areas of improvement identified through the BASICS chart. Ideally, the BASICS charts will identify areas of strength and areas for potential growth for each section of the curriculum. As students move through the curriculum, this process will help them become better self-reflective, self-monitoring students. To see an example of how to implement the BASICS chart, see Appendix A.

This guide is intended to assist readers through the transition of becoming a strength-based self-advocate. Professionals who work with people who have ASD can utilize the information presented in the text to facilitate discussions in a classroom setting, group setting, or individual meetings. Appendix B provides discussion points and questions that can be utilized by professionals as they see fit. The information presented is intended to be a starting point to be used with additional discussion, assignments, videos, etc. to best convey the information to specific student groups. Students using the text can take advantage of the reflection questions and worksheets to ensure a solid understanding of the topics presented. It is often the case that students benefit from consistent practice and consideration regarding new material and we have designed the text to reflect this notion. In addition, the information in this guide can be used as individuals work through the transition of becoming a self-advocate. Individuals can use this material and the guiding questions in Appendix B to move through this material independently or with support.

Individuals and professionals alike are encouraged to be creative with the material and to tailor it to their individual needs. While the material is written to provide knowledge and information about the positive qualities and strengths of individuals with ASD, there is no limit to the ways in which the material can be utilized within a specific context and this was intentional in our model. This guide is the result of research and was built on significant feedback from those college students with ASD who did not see their own strengths until after engaging in this work. As the true experts on ASD, these students have given us purpose and passion to help others with ASD see their own true potential in this world full of neurodiversity. We hope to provide our shared vision of opportunity and knowledge to individuals with ASD and those professionals who work with them during this exciting transition.

All worksheets marked with the symbol ⬇ are available for download from the JKP website at www.jkp.com/catalogue/book/9781849057974.

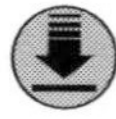

Table I.1 Back to BASICS Template

B	**Behavior** 1 2 3	**Comments**
A	**Academics** 1 2 3	**Comments**
S	**Self-care** 1 2 3	**Comments**
I	**Interaction** 1 2 3	**Comments**
C	**Community** 1 2 3	**Comments**
S	**Self-monitoring** 1 2 3	**Comments**

GOALS

Personal:

Academic:

Social:

Chapter 1

PERSONAL STORIES

There are no personal stories as powerful as the ones you tell about yourself.

INTRODUCTION

Our self-perception is shaped greatly by the stories people have told us about ourselves as we are growing up. Sometimes those stories are formed by how people treat us, while other times they can be formed by the things people say. Situations in your past that may seem like a small blip in your memory may in fact have lasting effects on how you view yourself. These personal stories begin forming as early as our memory can recall, often taking root in early childhood. This chapter will outline the potential impact people can have on self-perception. Each section will introduce portions of personal stories shared by people with ASD. The names and details have been changed but the themes of the memories are intact.

Our first impressions of ourselves come initially from our parents. Parents have a future vision of their children that is developed before the children are even born. Parents find out they are expecting a child and start imagining what their future child will become. They often think that their son will become a great doctor, actor, or recording artist. Their daughter will become the first female president, a professional athlete, or a teacher. However they imagine their child growing up, they typically picture them as perfect little versions of themselves who are emotionally connected and look at them with unconditional love and give hugs and kisses every day.

When that child is born with ASD, they may not have the same attachment to parents that neurotypical children have. Young children with ASD may not share the same level of physical contact and emotional connection with their parents, which is a very difficult thing for a parent to accept. Parents often blame themselves for not connecting with their children with ASD, which causes a lot of emotional strain on the family. In addition, parents may grieve the loss of the child they imagined and the type of relationship they see other parents having with their children. Children with ASD do not love their parents less, they simply have a different method of showing that love and the relationship is very different from what any parent imagines.

LESSON 1: EARLY CHILDHOOD

The following personal story reflects on the parent–child bond and how the difference made this person feel.

BOBBY'S STORY

"When I was not very old my mom would hug me a lot and I did not like it, and sometimes I would cry, but she would still hug me. I don't know why I didn't like it, but sometimes it would hurt. When I would fall and get hurt she would kiss me and I did not like that either, but she kept doing it. I did not understand why she would do this. Sometimes when I would pull away from my mom when she tried to hug me, she would cry. I didn't understand that either, but I didn't like to see my mom cry so I just let her hug and kiss me. I knew then that I didn't want to be the reason my mom was sad. I knew very young that I was different from most kids – but my mom didn't care, she just talked to me and taught me things. If someone was mean to me, she would stick up for me. She always protected me until I could do it myself."

How do you think this memory impacted Bobby's self-perception?

____

____

____

____

____

____

____

____

____

____

Other family members can also impact how we view ourselves. Siblings have been known to be mean to each other but also love and support one another. Grandparents typically love grandchildren immensely and unconditionally. Extended family looks very different from family to family. Some families are very close and share memories with aunts, uncles, and cousins while other families have relatives that they have never met. Regardless of how a family is formed, the memories of how family members engage inevitably impacts self-perception. Consider this following memory about how a family member impacted the personal story of this individual.

JOHN'S STORY

"I remember from a very early age that I spent a lot of time individually with my parents. Whether they were teaching me to use the bathroom, trying to get me to keep my clothes on, taking me to speech therapy, taking me to counseling, or trying to get me to read, it was always just me and my parents. I don't remember them spending time like that with my sister. She was only two years older than me, but she was so independent. She did everything by herself that I struggled to do with help. She always seemed so strong and smart, but now that I look back, she had to be. My parents were so wrapped up in supporting me that she had to grow up quickly. When I was about five years old she started being mean to me. She would punch me in the arm or pinch me when I sat by her. She would tell me I was weird and didn't want me to come into her room. She always told me to leave her alone. One time she told me that she hated me and wished I was never born."

How do you think this memory impacted John's self-perception?

____

____

____

____

____

____

____

____

____

____

People with ASD tend to have a lot of involvement with doctors. Medical doctors help manage the physical issues, psychologists help manage the emotional issues, and speech/language pathologists help with expressive and receptive language difficulties. All of these supports are positive and help the development of people with ASD; however, the language that is used in appointments can sometimes influence the way a person views him or herself. The professionals who have a primary function of helping people with ASD tend to have to start first with identifying areas that need improvement. As children go through the process of becoming diagnosed with ASD, many of these professionals engage in evaluations and discuss those findings with the parents. Sometimes the discussions about the diagnosis and reaction by the parents can stick in the memory and impact the way someone views themselves. Reflect on this memory shared by Susan about learning about her diagnosis at a young age.

SUSAN'S STORY

"I was diagnosed with autism many years ago. Not much was known about autism and at that time, parents often thought it was their fault that children were diagnosed. I remember going to so many appointments with different types of doctors who watched me and asked questions and watched me more. I didn't like the way they watched me. One day I was in the doctor's office with my mom and dad and the doctor told my mom and dad that I had autism and my mom started crying. I didn't know what autism was, but I remember thinking it must be bad if my mom is crying."

How do you think this memory impacted Susan's self-perception?

____

____

____

____

____

____

____

____

____

____

Another group of people that could have a significant impact on the development of self-perception is teachers. Teachers are with young children for multiple hours each day. They are tasked with teaching a group of children from a variety of backgrounds vital information that will help them develop into successful adults later in life. When students learn differently or have challenging needs, the relationship between teacher and student can be strained. Young children with ASD typically have not yet learned the coping strategies to be successful in the classroom so their behaviors can be a challenge in the large group setting. The interactions with a teacher can be very impactful in how a student with ASD views themselves as a learner. The following memory had a significant impact on Charlie.

CHARLIE'S STORY

"When I started school I got trouble nearly every day. I never really knew why I was in trouble, but teachers yelled at me and moved me to sit alone. I started each day telling myself that I wasn't going to get in trouble, but for some reason, I would get a headache and stomach ache after lunch. I didn't feel well so I would get cranky then I would get in trouble. The other kids stopped talking to me and didn't want to be around me. I loved recess because I could sit by the tree alone and just have quiet. I remember thinking there was something wrong with me when I was in first grade. When it was time to start second grade, I was so scared that I was going to get in trouble all the time again, but things were different. My teacher noticed early that I would start misbehaving after lunch. She talked with my mom and they started watching what I was eating. I found out that I was lactose intolerant and stopped eating dairy. My stomach felt better and I didn't get headaches as bad anymore. I didn't know why I was getting in trouble all the time, but my teacher figured it out."

How do you think this memory impacted Charlie's self-perception?

____

____

____

____

____

____

____

____

____

____

From the previous examples of personal stories from early childhood, you can see that any memory, big or small, can have an impact on how people with ASD view themselves. Take some time to reflect on your early childhood. Reach back as far as you can in your memory and write about the influence others had on your self-perception. You don't have to share this with anyone and it can be a great way to analyze how you formed your view of yourself. Be open and honest with your memories as they have contributed to your view of yourself.

Reflect on the story told to you by your parents:

Reflect on the story told to you by other family members:

Reflect on the story told to you by doctors:

Reflect on the story told to you by teachers:

LESSON 2: TEEN YEARS

Teen years are a difficult time to go through for everyone. Hormones are changing, bodies are changing, and relationships are changing. For people with ASD, all these changes make this time in life even more difficult to manage. As children, they would have found that the social rules were simple to learn and once learned, they didn't change much; however, the social rules change often in the teen years. People that were friends as children could enter into dating relationships, friends begin to "like" each other in different ways, style of dress and who you hang out with determines whether you are popular or weird, behaviors that were acceptable for children to do are no longer acceptable from a teen. For a child with ASD, this could be the most impactful time in the development of self-perception.

Everyone who has been through this developmental time can attest to the fact that teenagers can be mean. This is the time when bullying others who do not fit the social norm happens. Many people can talk about a time when they felt picked on or isolated because of something that made them stand out. Unfortunately, this happens all too often to teenagers who have ASD. Because middle school and high school are such social environments, people who struggle with understanding the social rules stand out and are often the victims of name calling and bullying. These difficult experiences can contribute significantly to a person's view of themselves and their view of ASD. It may become very difficult to remember strengths and talents while being bombarded with negative messages during these formative years. Lorie shares her memory of high school in the following excerpt of her personal story.

LORIE'S STORY

"The words used to describe me were usually 'nerd,' and 'geek.' There was a status system at school and I recognized I was firmly at the bottom of it. The athletes and cheerleaders were at the top, and the Dungeons and Dragons gamers were at the bottom. It wasn't that I didn't try to make friends; I desperately wanted friends, I just didn't know how to play by the same rules. I don't think I was even playing the same game. I remember being acutely aware of being the kid that people tried to avoid. The one who talked all the time about stuff that no one else understood, the object of people's jokes, and the owner of many horrible nicknames. I was the annoying kid that nobody wanted around. In high school, people have spots to sit for lunch with their groups. No groups wanted me at their tables so I tried to sit with the other social rejects, but even they didn't want me around."

How do you think this memory impacted Lorie's self-perception?

____

____

____

____

A significant change to the social world of teen years is the influx of social media. People easily become defined by how many "friends" they have on Facebook, how many "followers" they have on Instagram or how many "likes" they can get on a picture. Although "friends" on social media are not a genuine depiction of authentic friendships, unfortunately, teenagers' self-worth can become tied to the number of "friends" identified on the top of their home screen. College students have reported that social media is beginning to have a negative impact on the emotional health of users. This could be a direct result of the constant comparisons people engage in when their "friends" have more people following them, post pictures of them looking very good, share updates about how well they are doing in school, etc. The reality of the social media phenomena is that the people you follow are not accurate displays of who they really are. People will only post their best, not the areas with which they struggle. Consider the example given in Table 1.1:

Table 1.1 Virtual Stories

Social Media "Emma"	Real Life "Emma"
580 "friends" on Facebook	10 actual friends that she cares about
1,520 followers on Instagram	5 people that check in with her often
She gets 200 "likes" on pictures	She doesn't know the people liking her pictures
Pictures that show great grades	She has a math and writing tutor to help her get those grades
She posts "selfies" of her in a bikini	She desperately wants people to tell her she looks good because she doesn't have confidence in herself
She posts status updates about her plans for the weekend	She hopes that she will be invited to the party
She professes her love for her boyfriend	Her boyfriend is online and she hasn't met him in person

How do you think social media has impacted Emma's self-perception?

____

____

____

____

____

____

____

Community leaders, such as church leaders, school administrators, youth group organizers, and community recreation center supervisors can have an impact on the development of self-perception as well. Teens often look to this group of individuals for clarity when things become confusing in their lives. When people challenge their belief systems that have been present since childhood, teens will often look outside the family for guidance. The messages shared through words and actions from these leaders can have a lasting impact. Jeff shares a memory from his teen years that was particularly impactful.

JEFF'S STORY

"I was a part of our local youth group for most of my childhood and into my teen years. That was where I felt accepted and understood. I didn't feel like I had to perform, I could just be me and it was OK. One day I went to the youth group meeting and the director called my mom into the office. I wasn't invited in, but I could hear some of what he was saying. He told my mom that some of the parents were complaining about my behaviors and the kids were afraid of me. I ran outside at that point so I don't know what else was discussed, but I never went back to youth group again. I guess I messed up again."

How do you think this memory impacted Jeff's self-perception?

____

____

____

____

____

____

____

____

____

____

Again, from the examples of personal stories from teen years, you can see that any memory can have an impact on how people with ASD view themselves. Take some time to reflect on your teen years. Some memories may have been very positive, while others may be negative. Again, you don't have to share this with anyone and it can be a great way to analyze how you formed your view of yourself. Be open and honest with your memories as they have contributed to your view of yourself.

Reflect on the story told to you by peers during your teen years:

Reflect on the story you developed from the influence of social media:

Reflect on the story told to you by community leaders:

LESSON 3: YOUNG ADULTHOOD

As people enter young adulthood, many make the decision to attend college. This is a fresh start for people with ASD. They can begin a new chapter with different people who know very little about them. They can enter an environment that respects intellectual capacity at least as much as social capacity. People who thrive academically in college are well respected; they can choose to become socially involved or not, but they will not be judged by that level of involvement. There is a different set of social rules on a college campus, but everyone entering college must learn this new set of rules as well. This need to blend into the environment could also be a difficult task for people with ASD to manage.

Throughout the K–12 experience (educational experience prior to college), many students with ASD have been elevated by their academic ability. Their knowledge acquisition and performance have been their identity, but when they come to college, they are surrounded by thousands of people who thrive academically as well. Students may not stand out for this positive reason anymore and some students with ASD have voiced that they felt like they lost a part of their identity when they transitioned into college. They were no longer seen as "the smart one."

Research has told us that 43 percent of people diagnosed with ASD will attend post-secondary education (Chiang *et al.* 2012). This information supports the idea that this group of students is highly capable of academic success and the transition to the next level of education. This time in a young adult's life is when their view of the world, view of themselves, and belief systems are challenged. This is when their identity is being developed. They have a choice for the first time in their lives about who their friends are, what groups to join, and what classes to take. They are determining their own path, which can be both powerful and overwhelming.

The faculty in post-secondary education can have a lasting effect on the self-perception of students with ASD. Students who have always been the smartest kid in class, excellent in math, or high achieving in science may struggle with college level courses or may lack the executive functioning skills to stay abreast of all the requirements independently. The way in which a faculty member addresses these potential difficulties could have an immense impact on the self-perception of a person with ASD. Take, for example, the memory shared by Peter.

PETER'S STORY

"When I was in school, I was always the smart kid. I was the best in math and got all the math awards every year. That was my thing. Because I was so good at math, I decided I wanted to be an engineer so I could use my strength to create new technology. I was so excited and knew I was going to be successful in college. I got a really high ACT score in math so I was placed into a high-level math course my freshman year in college. I was confused from the very first day. I failed my first test and wanted to just hide in my room instead of going to college. I thought that if I wasn't good at even this math class, I was never going to be successful in college. Then my professor asked me to stay after class one day. I was terrified of what he was going to say to me, but it was a great meeting. He told me that I had the right ideas and he could tell I knew the material, but I was just missing a couple steps that involved thinking critically about a solution. I have never been asked to think critically about anything and that was really difficult, but when my professor told me it wasn't the mathematics part that was confusing me and offered to help with the part that I struggled with, I started doing much better in his class and felt better about the other classes as well. It was hard to admit that I needed help academically when I never needed it before."

How do you think this memory impacted Peter's self-perception?

____

____

____

____

____

____

____

____

____

____

Another relationship that will be new during this transition time is the relationship formed with roommates. Whether a student with ASD is living in a traditional residence hall sharing a bedroom and bathroom, or an apartment style residence hall, sharing a kitchen and living room, the act of sharing living space will be new. The process of communicating needs, difficulties, or disagreements appropriately is a skill that must be developed. The sensory needs, communication difficulties, and potential social confusion could make this process exponentially more difficult for college students with ASD. The process of self-disclosure to roommates is a personal decision and students must make those decisions about if and when to tell the roommates about ASD. In the event that the roommates do not accept this information well, a student's personal story could be negatively impacted. An example of this has been shared by Elise.

ELISE'S STORY

"The month before I moved from home to go to college in another town, I set up a meeting with my roommates and their families. My parents came as well and we all had dinner together. We had been communicating on Facebook for about a month so I felt like I knew them well enough to tell them that I have autism. We ate dinner and were chatting and I decided to tell them at the table about my diagnosis. I said that I have autism and sometimes I get very sensitive to loud noises and don't like to be patted. I also shared that I don't like cussing because I feel like it is wrong, but I can just put my ear plugs in anytime I need to. I thought I was doing the right thing, but then their parents told my parents that they needed to talk to her about the situation. I assume that meant that I was the situation because they left the table. After that, the girls didn't talk to me anymore and I just sat there alone. When my mom returned she was very upset and we left quickly. She told me that the parents told her they did not want their daughters to have to babysit me and that the girls thought I was weird anyway so they really didn't want me to room with them."

How do you think this memory impacted Elise's self-perception?

____

____

____

____

____

____

____

____

____

____

At this stage in development, people with ASD make several choices about their personal lives. Sometimes they choose to develop partnerships with classmates within the same major, or they choose to develop mentoring relationships with faculty, or some may choose to enter into intimate relationships with partners. This is often the first time a person with ASD has attempted this type of relationship and it can be quite intimidating. The rules associated with developing intimate relationships are confusing for neurotypical college students, but that confusion is heightened for students with ASD. Determining the level of the relationship, defining what level the intended relationship is, and picking up on the subtle social cues that the potential partner is giving can all be a source of anxiety, but if engaging in an intimate relationship is the choice, that chosen partner can be a source of positive or negative self-perception. Chris shared this memory of his first partner.

CHRIS' STORY

"I never really wanted to date in high school. It was all very confusing and there seemed to be a whole set of rules that everyone understood but were written in some foreign language to me. I heard people talking about me and they thought I was weird for not dating, but I just didn't feel ready. During my senior year in college, I decided I wanted to try dating but had no idea how to start to let someone know that I was interested. I had a girl in my class that was very attractive to me, but I didn't even know how to start a conversation with her. It was a research class so I decided to use the topic of the class to develop a compatibility test. I worked on the test for months, and then just before the class ended, I asked her to take part in my research project. She looked at me like I was the strangest person she had ever met, but she took the paper from me and walked out of class. She must have been intrigued because the very next class, she handed me the completed test. She asked me why I gave it to her to complete and I just blurted out that there was no denying that she was beautiful, but there was no point in asking her out if we were not compatible. She threw her head back and laughed so hard but then asked what the results were. I did some calculations and told her that according to my calculations we were 87 percent compatible so that means we should at least go have dinner. She agreed and we went on about six dates, but then she left for the summer and I graduated. She told me before she left that she had been asked out by a lot of guys, but she will always remember how I asked her out. We still talk occasionally."

How do you think this memory impacted Chris' self-perception?

Finally, from the examples of personal stories from young adulthood, you can see that any memory can have an impact on how people with ASD view themselves. Take some time to reflect on your young adulthood, beginning with college years if this is in the past for you. Some memories may have been very positive, while others may be difficult to think about, but all of them have had an impact. Again, you don't have to share this with anyone and it can be a great way to analyze how you formed your view of yourself. Be open and honest with your memories as they have contributed to your view of yourself.

Reflect on the story told to you by faculty members in college:

Reflect on the story told to you by roommates:

Reflect on the story told to you by a partner:

____

____

____

____

____

____

____

____

____

____

____

____

The process of reflecting on how others have treated us and how that has impacted our own development is a very difficult process. The recognition that people have not always treated us with the level of respect we would hope for can be emotional but can also give us a glimpse into how we have formulated our own self-concept. Neurotypical people tend to be more impacted by the subtle messages and behaviors displayed by others, but there is no denying that people with ASD have also allowed others to write their own personal stories. Whether it was a bully in elementary school, a doctor who talked too much about deficits, a community leader who disengaged, or a college roommate who didn't want to share a living environment, all too often, the power of writing personal stories has been surrendered to other people.

LESSON 4: WRITING YOUR OWN STORY

At this point in development, the time has come to take the power back and write your own story. What do you want others to recognize about you? How do you want people to perceive you? How do you want to view yourself? By recognizing what you have learned from others throughout your life, you can find the power to write your own personal story.

WRITE YOUR OWN STORY

Main character description:

____

____

____

____

____

____

Main character's strengths:

____

____

____

____

____

____

Main character's nemesis:

____

____

____

____

____

____

Plot twist:

Conflict resolution:

Your main character's contribution to the world:

____

____

____

____

____

____

____

____

____

____

____

____

____

This chapter has allowed you to examine the impact others have had on your personal stories as you have grown up. These stories may have been words said to you, looks given to you, or the way people have treated you. You have been given the opportunity to become the author of your own personal story making yourself the main character. This is the first step in revising how you view yourself as a person with ASD. Moving forward, you will be encouraged to start viewing yourself through a different lens: a lens that is more positive and reflective of strengths. Only you can control how you feel about yourself and how you regard yourself and others with ASD. This first step of rewriting your own story is vital, so keep this story in focus as you work through this guide and start celebrating your role in the ASD community. Take some time to reflect on the work you have done in this chapter and rate yourself honestly using the BASICS chart. This self-evaluation can help guide your development throughout this book.

BACK TO BASICS

Consider these guiding questions as you prepare to evaluate yourself.

B	**Behavior**	How do you tell your personal stories? Are you aware of their impact on other people? What are your reactions to the personal stories of others? Are you responding well to remembering details in your personal stories? Are you considering when you might disclose ASD?
A	**Academics**	Are you attending all your classes on time? Are you applying organizational strategies? What are you saying about your organizational system? Are you keeping up with everything?
S	**Self-care**	Are you getting enough sleep? Are you eating healthily? Are you planning for your self-care activities? Are you keeping your space clean? What are you doing to make sure you are managing your stress level?
I	**Interaction**	Are you checking in with your support team? Are you planning time for social activities? Are you actively engaged in classes? What are you doing to get to know your roommates? Are you checking your email/blackboard daily?
C	**Community**	Do you feel like you belong? Are you asking for help when needed? Have you met anyone new? Do you know the names of any classmates? Are you involved in anything socially?
S	**Self-monitoring**	Are you managing your time? Are you accepting critical feedback? Are you managing your frustration level? Are you willing to see the perspectives of others? Are you advocating for yourself?

BACK TO BASICS: RATE YOURSELF

B	**Behavior** 1 2 3	**Comments**
A	**Academics** 1 2 3	**Comments**
S	**Self-care** 1 2 3	**Comments**
I	**Interaction** 1 2 3	**Comments**
C	**Community** 1 2 3	**Comments**
S	**Self-monitoring** 1 2 3	**Comments**

GOALS

Personal:

Academic:

Social:

Chapter 2

THE LANGUAGE OF ASD

The power of words can hurt or help a person's self-perception.

INTRODUCTION

Universities and colleges, both public and private, are microcosms of their regions and communities, bringing many different populations together for higher education. For some students, this might mean interacting with people of a different race or someone who primarily speaks a different language. For others, it can be their most authentic exposure yet to hierarchies of socio-economic status or issues of privilege in gender. As with other variations in the college student and community populations, disability is factored into the assessment of diversity. There is certainly a sense that, in addition to facilitating academic curricula and the development of innovative research and scholarship, college is a unique setting also charged with fostering holistic student identities.

When we consider identity development as an element of the college experience, we can use the basic premise of James Marcia's theory of identity development to introduce our discussion of the comparisons between identity language and diagnostic language (Marcia 2002). Marcia's work suggests that identity in adolescents is developed through crisis, in which an individual is reconsidering existing values and personal choices, and commitment, occurring through choices, role, or identity. College, traditionally the setting in which an adolescent might be re-evaluating values and choices upon newfound independence, is, for many students, an environment fostering commitment to choices, values, and roles. When one has a strong sense of self, produced through their commitment to choices and values, strength recognition is evident. It is when lack of identity persists that individual strength and challenges are unknown. Assuming most college students are engaged in some way in the development of values and identity, the presence of student organizations, diversity-directed support staff and programming, and student-initiated events and groups are no surprise. These diverse groups serve as places of social research for those students who might be considering their values and making new or different choices in their lives. They are also places of learning, growth, and camaraderie for those sharing common identity elements or values.

Diversity on college campuses, then, is abundantly displayed. College students identifying with diverse groups gather with those who are like-minded to share ideas and common experiences. Entire student support services funded through universities or even federal grants and mandates are geared toward student identities. Women's centers, multicultural centers, lesbian, gay, bisexual, and transgender (LGBT) student support resources, international student services, disability resources, campus athletics, and student leadership initiatives can be found on most campuses, providing direct resources for those who have identified with diverse identifying groups. Not all student groups are staffed by university personnel with designated spaces; some are led by students and driven by student interests. Student organizations are indicative of the diverse values that students have at college. For instance, students may take part in campus religious programs, student government groups, an array of advocacy organizations for passions of all kinds, or intramural sports. Discussions about identity in the college environment allow us to connect to the notion that identity is fostered in this setting perhaps more than any other for those who choose to pursue higher education, where diversity is prevalent and largely celebrated.

LESSON 1: IDENTITY MODELS

Before we go on to examine language that students associate with autism, the concept of neurodiversity can help us understand what identity can mean for college students with autism. Essentially, neurodiversity suggests that differences in human brains can be attributed simply to natural variation. Advocates of neurodiversity understand autism and other disabilities such as Attention Deficit Hyperactivity Disorder (ADHD) and dyslexia through a lens that filters out social prejudice and language used in deficit models. Differences in a neurodiverse world are products of genetic predisposition and environment, settling, at least in this context, debates of nature versus nurture. It is this view that argues that individuals, especially those with ASD, who have unconventionally unique brains, are not broken and need no cure, but rather actively provide society with some important and distinctive benefits in a general world sense. Neurodiversity and its impact increase on campuses as the number of students with autism and other diagnoses like ADHD entering institutions of higher education increases.

Unlike when we consider positive changes in attitudes about issues of race, gender, and sexuality, understanding a disability like autism involves not only these positive societal changes, but recognizing a functional reality as well. Diagnostic language by its very nature emphasizes labels, but it can give a welcome sense of understanding when there might otherwise exist only confusion. It is with language that reframes this jargon into positive and very real identity factors that we allow for the validation and celebration of the strengths and differences inherent in people with ASD. Focusing on a cure or attempting to change or diminish idiosyncrasies in a population of college students in the crux of identity development lessens the opportunity for society to celebrate differences in the ways of thinking that have certainly been fundamental to our life experiences and extensive world knowledge. While it is true that individuals on the spectrum might be impacted in an array of daily functions, from planning a project to engaging in small talk on the elevator, the concept of neurodiversity allows us to include the symptoms of autism with factors of identity that, when committed to and reframed, can promote strengths instead of deficits and advantages instead of limitations.

To demonstrate the way the diagnostic model and neurodiversity model explain disability, the next exercise will challenge you to reflect on your experiences with both models. We use brain imagery not to suggest that the elements listed are necessarily relative to the colored area, but to show that these models do not rely on information about any demographic group. In fact, with this image there is little opportunity for bias when we consider the bare information represented by the image. All we can see is the brain; we do not see gender, age, race, religion, or any other element.

These models can convey quite distinctive attitudes about people with disabilities. The focus of these models is based solely on how you as an individual with ASD view the impact of ASD. It is clear that reframing your view in any of these areas can in fact promote more recognition of strengths and ability rather than focusing on deficits.

COMPARING LANGUAGE MODELS

Examine the elements of language, focus, identity, message, and goal of each of the two models. Then, using the empty image, fill in each area with your own experiences with the elements of each model. Fill in the information for how you may view yourself through a diagnostic lens, and then redirect your thoughts and fill in the information for how you view yourself through a neurodiversity lens.

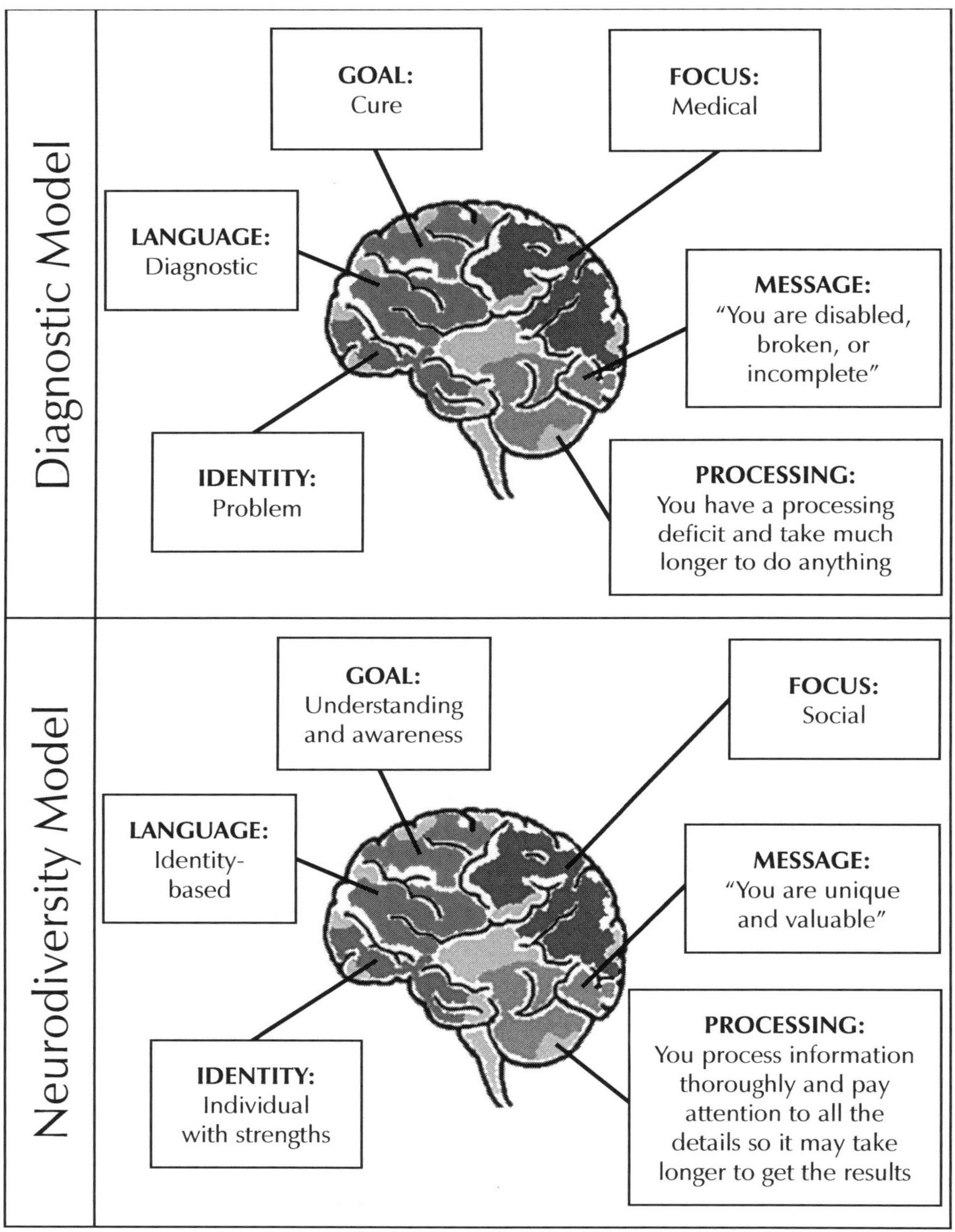
Diagnostic Model
GOAL: Cure
FOCUS: Medical
LANGUAGE: Diagnostic
MESSAGE: "You are disabled, broken, or incomplete"
IDENTITY: Problem
PROCESSING: You have a processing deficit and take much longer to do anything
Neurodiversity Model
GOAL: Understanding and awareness
FOCUS: Social
LANGUAGE: Identity-based
MESSAGE: "You are unique and valuable"
IDENTITY: Individual with strengths
PROCESSING: You process information thoroughly and pay attention to all the details so it may take longer to get the results

FIGURE 2.1: DIAGNOSTIC VS. NEURODIVERSITY IMPACT ON THINKING

Complete each box with experiences and thoughts from your own life within each of these models.

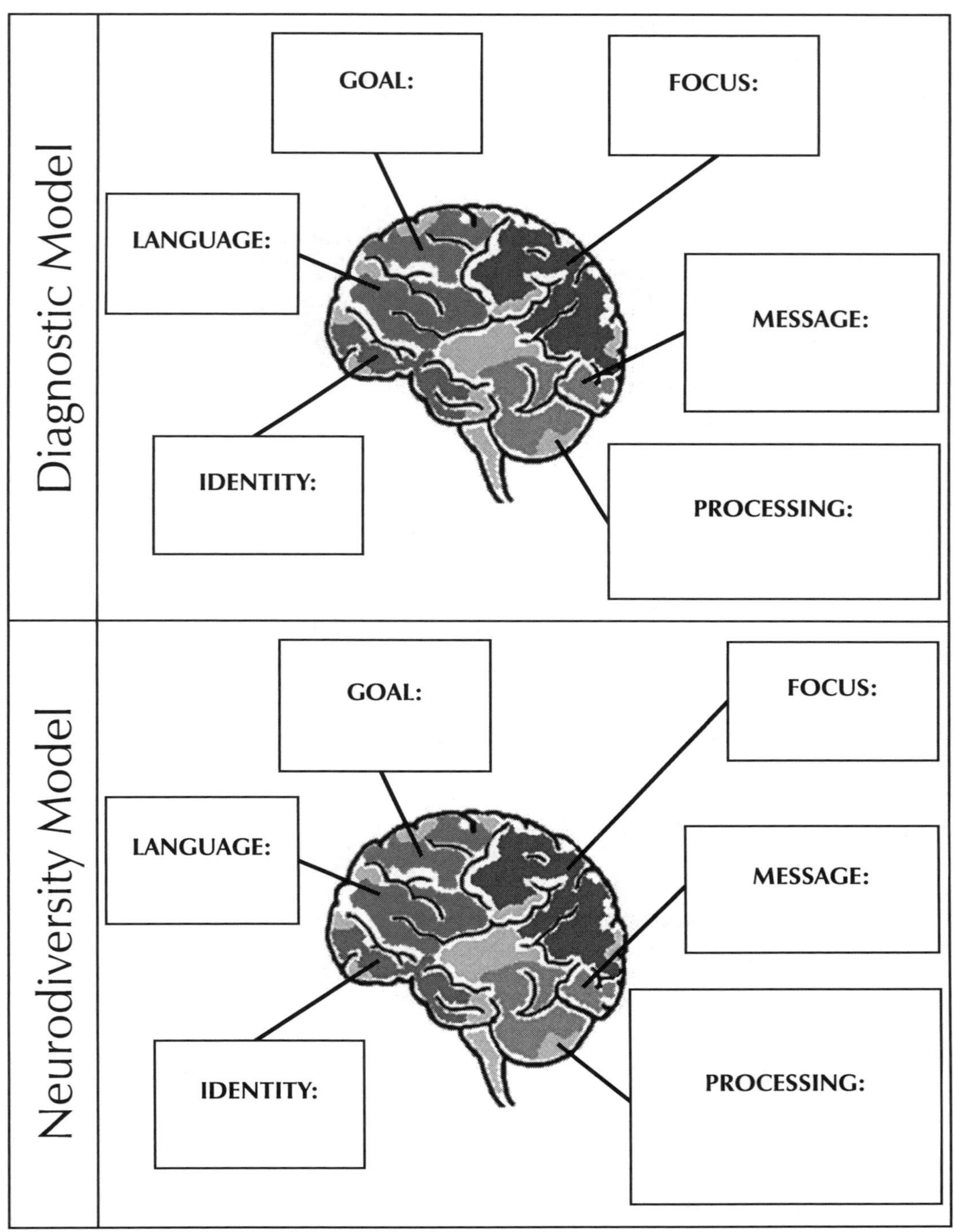

LESSON 2: DIAGNOSTIC LANGUAGE

People diagnosed with ASD all share a similar experience of going through the evaluation process for ASD and hearing the resulting findings. Regardless of the diagnostic tools used, the language in the majority of these tools is similarly negative. The focus of diagnostic language serves a purpose but can also contribute to the development of negative self-perceptions.

To diagnose a person with ASD, a qualified professional must meet with the individual, family members, educators, and anyone else who can contribute to the personal story of the individual being evaluated. Often, these stories are filled with all the behavioral difficulties from early childhood, the difficulty with staying focused, the deficits in language development, the inability to fit in socially, and the restricted interests. The purpose behind the diagnostic language is to highlight the difficulties to gain an understanding of the level of impact the diagnosis is having on the individual, but the discussion of the diagnosis can be done in a much more positive way.

Although these pieces of information are vital in gaining a diagnosis that could offer positive benefits, if not discussed responsibly in the presence of the person being diagnosed, the negative effects could be lasting. If an individual does receive a formal diagnosis of ASD, he or she could gain access to the necessary therapies and support needed to develop strategies for a successful and productive life. If the diagnosis is not discussed appropriately in front of the individual, the therapies may have to begin with reversing the influence of the language on the self-perception of the individual. This negative impression could be a constant reminder of the fact that they are not "normal."

Some of the diagnostic language used in many evaluative tools can be interpreted as follows:

- Persistent deficit
- Disadvantage
- Underdeveloped social skills
- Lack of non-verbal understanding
- Ritualized patterns of behavior
- Insistence on sameness
- Failure to develop appropriate relationships
- Insufficiencies in maintaining relationships
- Stereotyped behaviors
- Obsessive interest in unusual topics
- Over/under-reactivity to environmental factors
- Lack of understanding of social cues
- Poor social communication

- Clinically significant impairment
- Disturbances
- Interests abnormal in intensity for age
- Delayed or undeveloped speech

BRAINSTORMING THE PERCEPTIONS OF OTHERS

As a person with ASD, you may have heard some of these words used to describe you or your diagnosis previously. After reading back through the diagnostic language, reflect on words that come to mind to describe you as a person with ASD. For five minutes, write the words that come to mind in the speech bubble below.

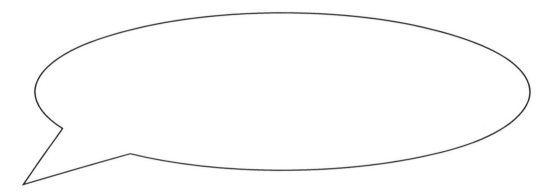

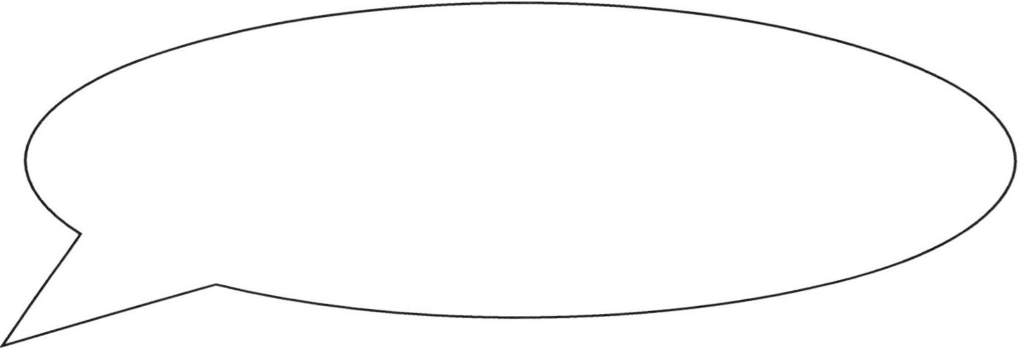

In developing this guide, previous college students with ASD were asked the same question. After gathering the thoughts of many college students with ASD who spent five minutes writing to describe themselves, the following word cloud was developed. The words in this word cloud are honest representations of how the students viewed themselves at the time. Identify any words that are similar to your list in the previous speech bubble.

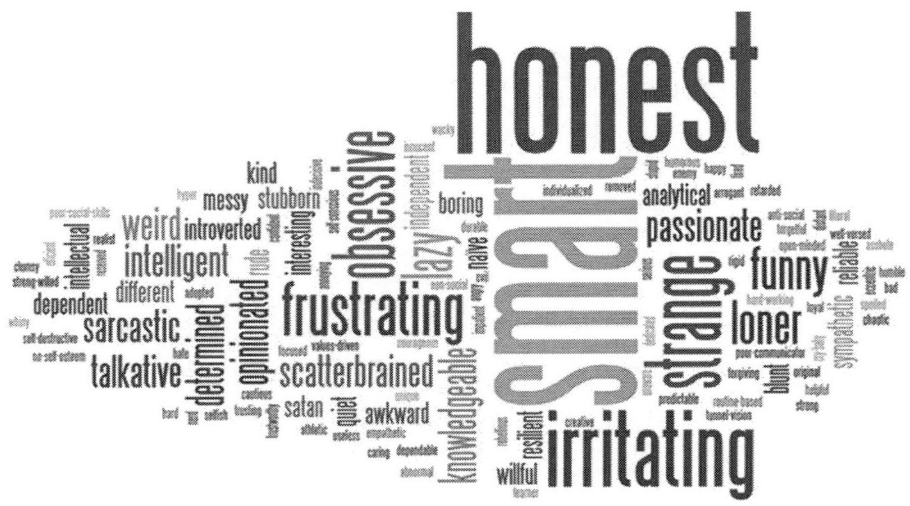

FIGURE 2.3

LESSON 3: IDENTITY LANGUAGE

Throughout development, young adults frequently come into contact with people or experiences that help shape their personal identities. Whether joining an Honors Program for academic and scholarly excellence or joining a service-based fraternity to build a professional network, individuals seek out people who share similar characteristics and interests. It is these characteristics and interests that shape how young adults define themselves as they develop into adulthood.

Far too frequently individuals develop their identities based on how others have defined them. Perhaps in high school, others define a girl as the popular girl. This identity definition determines how she interacts with others, experiences educational activities, and ultimately how she perceives herself among her peers. Perhaps that same girl is defined by others as the brainiac. This identity definition could completely change how she experiences her high school years. She may study instead of going out with friends, she may join the Beta Club instead of becoming a cheerleader, and she may view herself in relation to her peers very differently despite the fact that she is the same person. These titles and the accompanying self-perceptions tend to stick with individuals until their personal identity is redefined through exposure to new ways of thinking about themselves.

Carrying any identity title can have its own inherent stressors, but the related stress can be managed if the individual is creating their own title based on how their individual identity is defined. If you define your own strength and identity you will be able to take ownership and this will then be likely to become a more protected and celebrated part of you. This idea of creating identity can be expanded to include identifying positively as a person with ASD. To help alleviate the negative emotion associated with an autism diagnosis, the following Identity Criteria have been developed (Atwood 1999). To be able to identify as a person with ASD, you must:

- Be a strong thinker
- Recognize persistent advantages of ASD
- Have high-quality social relationships
- Have relationships free of manipulation
- Have relationships based on shared interests and values
- Be honest in relationships
- Feel safe when things are predictable
- Be consistent
- Demonstrate individualized and creative behaviors
- Be highly intelligent about specific topics
- Be in tune with environment

- Take people at face value
- Offer authentic communication in interactions with others
- Understand your strengths
- Be able to relate well to those who are younger or older
- Have a strong grasp of vocabulary.

DIAGNOSTIC LANGUAGE VS. IDENTITY CRITERIA

To better understand the concept of Diagnostic vs. Identity-based ways of living your life as a person with ASD, consider the following chart. The words used in the Diagnostic Language section are actual words used to diagnose someone with ASD; the words used in the Identity Criteria section are the same message, but use different wording. Attribute each word to you as a person with ASD and share how that word makes you view yourself.

Diagnostic Language	Response	Identity Criteria	Response
• Persistent deficit		• Strength of thought	
• Underdeveloped social skills		• High-quality social relationships	
• Lack of non-verbal understanding		• Relationships free of manipulation	
• Over/under-reactivity to environmental factors		• In tune with environmental factors	
• Ritualized patterns of behavior		• Predictability	
• Insistence on sameness		• Consistency	
• Failure to develop appropriate relationships		• Relationships based on shared interests/ values	
• Obsessive interests		• Highly intelligent	
• Lack of understanding of social cues		• Takes people at face value	
• Delayed speech		• Strong vocabulary	

LESSON 4: DIAGNOSTIC CRITERIA AND THE IMPACT ON COMMUNITY

Diagnostic manuals are based on the current research and best practices established in the field. These tools are periodically reviewed and revised based on the feedback from practitioners, updated research, newly developed criteria, etc. When these revisions occur, it is plausible that the definition of various disability types will be completely rewritten. During these revisions, new criteria are established which could result in subtypes of disabilities being completely removed from the diagnostic manual. While respected clinicians and groups of scientific researchers work together to review and revise these manuals, little attention is given to the potential impact on the sense of community established within people who identify with the particular disability subtypes.

An example of this impact is the revision to the *Diagnostic and Statistical Manual of Mental Disorders* forming the current version, *DSM-5* (American Psychiatric Association 2013). Noted experts in the field and scientific researchers gathered and worked through potential revisions for nearly a decade. Criteria for the many identified disorders in the manual were studied and discussed and new criteria were established for many of these disorders. Through this process the diagnosis of Asperger's Syndrome was essentially eliminated as a subtype. Although it will remain intact for those who already have this established diagnosis, the label Asperger's Syndrome is no longer evident in the diagnostic manual. Instead of the previous set of subtypes of autism, all subtypes were lumped together under Autism Spectrum Disorder and the distinction between them was defined by severity instead of subtype title. This created intense controversy among the "Aspie" community because the established diagnostic label was the umbrella that established the sense of community.

Because of the importance to the community of the label within the diagnostic manual, this community of like-minded, strong, and unique individuals was essentially left without a sense of place. According to the diagnostic language, they no longer fit anywhere. This group that had established a new set of norms and culture that focused on strengths and the qualities of "Aspies" that were to be celebrated was deleted from existence. Although people who would qualify as having Asperger's could still qualify under the new version, they seemed to have lost their identity with the label. The qualities that set them apart from others are still there, but they no longer have the diagnostic label.

By adopting the Identity Criteria in place of Diagnostic Criteria, you can hold on to your sense of community while celebrating your shared diverse way of interacting with the world. By taking the approach of including ASD within your personal identity, no matter how many times the diagnostic manuals are revised, no matter how many times the label ASD is changed, your sense of self and personal identity can remain intact.

Describe what makes up your personal identity:

LESSON 5: OWNING ASD

Once an individual with ASD has accepted and included ASD as a part of his or her identity, the process moves to truly embracing and owning the qualities of ASD as a part of the individual. The focus up until now has been heavily steered toward developing an understanding that there are significant strengths associated with ASD, but there is no denying that there are some difficulties inherent in ASD as well. The empowering piece of understanding these difficulties is being able to disclose, educate, discuss, and problem-solve around those difficulties before they become a problem in relationships. This puts the individual with ASD in control of the experiences he or she encounters. The individual can become the driver in the interactions before the relationship becomes difficult.

Take for example, a college student with ASD moving into a residence hall on a college campus. This young adult has advocated for establishing a need for a private bedroom within the suite-style residence hall, but will need to be able to share a bathroom, kitchen, and living room with three other young adults. Now imagine that this young adult is you. What potential difficulties could arise if you did not engage in a conversation with roommates about your habits and specific needs?

____

____

____

____

____

____

____

____

____

____

Use this following script as an example for how a disclosure conversation with a college roommate could proceed.

> "I know our roommate contract discussion is a time to talk about the things we need in our living environment and I think it is a good time to tell you all about some things I do differently. I have an Autism Spectrum Disorder, which means that I process things differently. I am very sensitive to sound so I will probably be wearing headphones a lot. I also am very protective of my personal space and things, so I would really appreciate it if you didn't use my things without asking.

> One thing that I am working on, but still struggle with, is that I am often very blunt and honest. Sometimes that comes across as rude, but that is not my intention. If I say something that offends you, please tell me so I can learn to manage this part of my personality. There are other things that I do differently, but I would be happy to talk about them as they come up. Please ask any questions you have and don't be afraid to talk with me about anything that may concern you."

Now write your own script to help you disclose ASD to a potential roommate. Keep in mind all of the things that are important to you and the things that may cause strife with someone.

____

____

____

____

____

____

____

____

____

____

____

____

____

____

____

____

____

Another group of people that could benefit from truly understanding how you process information and interact with others is the group of college professors with whom you may interact frequently. Without understanding the impact ASD may have on your daily interactions, a professor could potentially view you as an arrogant student who tries to prove the professor wrong or the student that hijacks the classroom conversation to show off. The following script could be used to disclose ASD to your professor.

"Dr. Smith, I just wanted to take a minute to talk with you about something that could impact how we interact in the classroom. I have an Autism Spectrum Disorder and because of that I sometimes have a difficult time understanding social cues. In the classroom, I may take over a conversation and not even recognize that you are trying to get me to stop talking. I hope to control my talking to only three times during our class meeting times. If I have follow-up questions, I will try to email you quickly. I also get very engaged in conversations about topics that I really love and sometimes it can come across as if I am trying to prove to people that my perspective is correct. It is not meant to be rude; I just get very excited about certain topics. If you could just let me know if I speak too much or come across as disrespectful, I can work on developing the skills to control this. If you ever have any questions or want to talk with me about this, I would be happy to talk to you about it."

Now write your own script for disclosing ASD to a professor to avoid any potential conflicts in the classroom.

____

____

____

____

____

____

____

____

____

____

____

____

____

____

____

In this chapter, you have had the opportunity to see the impact of diagnostic language and the impact of creating your identity that includes ASD as a part of your personhood. Owning ASD and embracing all the inherent strengths that come along with that part of your identity may help you develop into a strong, secure self-advocate, a self-advocate who can not only display strengths and educate about the positive features of ASD, but can also recognize your needs and build a support system in your environment to ensure your own success. By discussing your strengths and potential pitfalls with people in your support system, you can have the opportunity to be yourself while learning new strategies to avoid social miscues.

Reflect on the impact diagnostic language has had on your view of yourself. In addition, think about the possibility of shifting your view and completely embracing ASD as a part of your identity that should be celebrated. Use the BASICS chart to honestly evaluate your growth in this area. By considering the areas in which you may still struggle, you can become a self-evaluating learner and guide your further development.

BACK TO BASICS

Consider these guiding questions as you prepare to evaluate yourself.

B	**Behavior**	How do you respond to diagnostic language? Are you comfortable using identity language? What are your reactions to diagnostic language changes? Are you connecting with your ASD community? Are you confident in owning ASD?
A	**Academics**	Are you attending all your classes on time? Are you applying organizational strategies? Are you consistently using your organizational system? Are you keeping up with everything?
S	**Self-care**	Are you getting enough sleep? Are you eating healthily? Are you planning for your self-care activities? Are you keeping your space clean? What are you doing to make sure you are managing your stress level?
I	**Interaction**	Are you checking in with your support team? Are you planning time for social activities? Are you actively engaged in classes? What are you doing to get to know your roommates? Are you checking your email/blackboard daily?
C	**Community**	Do you feel like you belong? Are you asking for help when needed? Have you met anyone new? Do you know the names of any classmates? Are you involved in anything socially?
S	**Self-monitoring**	Are you managing your time? Are you accepting critical feedback? Are you managing your frustration level? Are you willing to see the perspectives of others? Are you advocating for yourself?

BACK TO BASICS: RATE YOURSELF

B	**Behavior** 1 2 3	**Comments**
A	**Academics** 1 2 3	**Comments**
S	**Self-care** 1 2 3	**Comments**
I	**Interaction** 1 2 3	**Comments**
C	**Community** 1 2 3	**Comments**
S	**Self-monitoring** 1 2 3	**Comments**

GOALS

Personal:

Academic:

Social:

Chapter 3

ASD IN THE MEDIA

Don't let what others portray in the media be your truth.

INTRODUCTION

As we learned in the previous chapter, young adulthood is about finding out who you are, developing your own beliefs and values system, and understanding how to identify with the world around you. More simply put, this is the time when young adults develop their worldview. Our worldviews are shaped by life experiences, education, exposure to different things, and what we hear from reliable sources. Often, those reliable sources include the media. More often than not young adults gather information from some form of media source and form opinions based on what the media tells them to believe. Whether they read the *New York Times* every morning, scroll through Facebook clicking on things that look interesting, or listen to peers talk about their perspectives on current events, young adults are developing opinions on the subject matter and shaping how they perceive what is happening in the world around them.

People with ASD tend to form their opinions based on knowledge acquisition from various sources so their worldview may not be as easily shaped by the media, but it is important to remember that others place significant importance on the information presented through media resources. Society sometimes forms perceptions based on information presented and interpreted differently by the viewers. This skewed potential perception may reinforce the inappropriate and often misguided perception that people with ASD are dangerous. People with ASD, advocates, and viewers have a much bigger role in how we choose to filter information, project responses, and process the effects that the media has on our views.

As technology has become a major part of our lives so has the way we receive and sometimes even process information. Throughout the last decade we have seen ASD through the lens of television shows, news sources, research, journals, and of course social media. Previously, stories in the media often painted a picture of individuals with ASD as broken or dangerous. More recently society as a whole has pushed for a more positive approach by advocating and educating people regarding the actuality of the impact of ASD. Whether or not they are portraying positive or negative perceptions, the media can have long-lasting effects on how ASD is viewed globally.

In Temple Grandin's book *The Way I See It* (2011) she talks about disability vs. behavior issues. She explains that some types of behavior are not necessary disability-related but are results of not understanding the needs in one's environment. In recent news coverage, we are starting to see the same shift. Professionals, news anchors, and writers are discussing comorbidity and potential underlying mental health issues when ASD has a questionable link to a current event. Instead of automatically attributing a violent event to ASD, reporters are actively discussing other potential causes for the event. As we see this shift in ASD awareness, the media is beginning to respond appropriately. It is the responsibility of viewers to continue this push for realistic and accurate reporting to cause no further harm to the reputation of people in the ASD community.

LESSON 1: DEVELOPMENT OF PERCEPTIONS THROUGH POPULAR MEDIA

As students begin to recognize the impact that popular media can have on the perception of people with ASD, it is first important to understand why others tend to allow their perceptions of an entire population to be defined by the actions of a few people. Many times, this is due to the lack of understanding of ASD. Because people with ASD are largely misunderstood and there is no definitive set of characteristics of the population of people with ASD, it is easy for people who don't understand to create their own stories. Often when people create their own stories, they will be drama-filled and much worse. This propensity to be guided by others can be shifted if self-advocates develop the inner strength to do appropriate educating about people with ASD. The first step is to develop an understanding of how messages get clouded in the media.

These messages can be processed very differently by people with ASD and people who are neurotypical. These messages can also be interpreted and perceived differently among the population of people with ASD. Consider how you perceive the messages you see and hear through the media as a person with ASD as compared to someone who is not on the spectrum.

PROCESSING THE IMPACT OF THE MEDIA

Use the following images to summarize a news story about a person with ASD. Below, reflect on the story and discuss it with someone who has less knowledge of ASD than you, and who can give you insight into how they have processed the information. On the next image, document how you processed the information along with how another person with less knowledge about ASD processed this same information.

MESSAGE PROCESSED BY YOU

What people see in the media:	What message do you develop about ASD?
____________________	____________________
____________________	____________________
____________________	____________________
____________________	____________________
____________________	____________________
____________________	____________________
____________________	____________________
____________________	____________________
____________________	____________________

MESSAGE PROCESSED BY OTHERS

What people see in the media:

____
____
____
____
____
____
____
____
____

What message do you develop about ASD?

____
____
____
____
____
____
____
____
____

LESSON 2: ASD IN THE NEWS

The general public often believes what they see, hear, or read in what they view as reliable sources. Information is easily accessible and people are quick to assume. Any current event is reported on through several media outlets. Anytime something in the world happens, that information can be found by turning on the television or simply doing a search to find it online. Because of the significant competition in journalism, news agencies are quick to get a jump on the other sources when events happen. This desire to be the first to report cutting-edge, attention-seeking stories could contribute to uninformed speculation or information that is not presented entirely accurately. Although some stories can be very uplifting and encouraging, it is unfortunate that many news stories are doom-and-gloom types of stories that focus on the negative experiences of humanity.

For example, there have been several stories reported throughout the past several years about the horrendous things that have happened at elementary schools, airports, movie theatres, and universities. Many of the stories in the media have tried to loosely tie the atrocities to people with ASD. Although the tie to ASD is a stretch at best, this negative connection can be detrimental when someone has very little knowledge of ASD. Another potential effect of the impact of reporting information that is not completely factual is the premise that environmental factors or parental decisions could be the cause of ASD. We most recently were witness to a line of reporting in which a well-known television personality made the claim that the mercury in vaccines was the cause of her son's autism diagnosis. The effect of this irresponsible reporting was evident when parents of children diagnosed with ASD refrained from vaccinating their children against many childhood illnesses. It wasn't until years later that the doctor from this story was proven wrong, but that took away years of media attention that could have been reporting more educational content.

ANALYZING THE MESSAGE IN THE MEDIA

To be able to combat what you hear in the news, you have to first be educated about what people are saying. Whether the reports are positive or negative, you must be a diligent viewer and arrive at your own conclusions. Only then can you truly be an education self-advocate who can combat the negative stereotypes presented through the media. Conduct a search for ASD in the media and find no less than three sources and report the following information:

- News source
- Important information in the report
- Connection with ASD
- Positive or negative connection
- Whether the connection is based on fact or is for dramatic effect
- How you can use this information to educate about ASD.

Source 1:

Source 2:

Source 3:

As an active member of the ASD community, it becomes your role to advocate for the accurate representation of people on the spectrum. Develop and discuss a plan for how you can become an educational advocate about the realities of ASD to negate reports in the media. How can you use this information to help others understand negative reporting and the accurate information related to ASD?

LESSON 3: ASD IN MOVIES AND TELEVISION

In 2010, Temple Grandin shared her story with the world and opened the eyes of millions in her HBO movie titled *Temple Grandin.* In this movie, Claire Danes portrayed Temple very accurately and showed a life of difficulty but a person with perseverance who pushed through the adversity of an early diagnosis, turbulent high school years, and was helped by a science teacher (Roybal 2008; Wallis 2010). Temple went on to become a well-known doctor of animal science, college professor, and autism activist. Unlike other movies that portray individuals with ASD, this movie was correct in its depiction of Temple Grandin (Royal 2008; Wallis 2010).

Other movies make attempts at attributing ASD qualities to main characters, but do so in a dramatic way to gain more viewers. While this creates a higher level of entertainment value, the inherent inaccuracies create stereotypical understanding of ASD. For example, in 1998, Dustin Hoffman starred in the movie *Rain Man.* In this movie, his character was portrayed as an individual with ASD but displayed characteristics more in line with that of Savant Syndrome. His character was able to count cards accurately, count spilled matchsticks, and calculate almost instantaneously the number left in the box, but could not carry on a meaningful conversation. He reacted violently to unexpected noises and did not display age-appropriate responses to interactions. These characteristics may be aligned with the characteristics of a savant; however, they are not necessarily accurate for ASD in general. People who do not know much about ASD could interpret that behavior as typical for this population and develop unnecessary fear of this population based on the behaviors displayed by this character.

The same difficulties can be discussed when viewing television characters with characteristics of ASD. One of the most well-known characters that display ASD qualities is Dr. Sheldon Cooper in *The Big Bang Theory.* Writers continue to conceal whether they in fact intended for Sheldon to be a character with ASD. The experiences of Sheldon continue to display accurate characteristics of someone living successfully with ASD. They do not hide the fact that Sheldon struggles socially and has many rituals that he must stick with to maintain control of his life. These are displayed routinely in episode after episode, but the writers still avoid giving credence to this claim. Perhaps the weight of displaying ASD characteristics accurately and responsibly would take away from the creativity, or the stigma attached to labeling a character could take away from the storyline, or a number of other possibilities exist for why they choose not to attach the diagnosis to this character, but despite the lack of commitment to the formality of the diagnosis, the writers do continue to provide an accurate picture of how some of the characteristics of ASD may appear in social and occupational settings.

There are many other characters in movies and in television that display some of the qualities associated with ASD. Some are accurate while others send a mixed picture of the reality of living with ASD mixed with the Hollywood hype of dramatization to make a character conflict-filled or more lovable than reality would present. By having a clear understanding of the genuine qualities of ASD, you may be able to develop an affinity for characters presented in movies or television. You don't have to share all qualities, but you may be able to relate.

LESSON 4: ASD IN SOCIAL MEDIA

Social media has recently become the way most young adults get the news of the day. Whether you are following news sources on Twitter, following what is trending on Facebook, watching podcasts on YouTube, or monitoring recent practices through Tumblr, this outlet of information is replacing newspapers and television news sources. People get the information in small bites very quickly through these sites and don't have to use too much of their time to stay up to date on current events. Unfortunately, there is a negative side effect of this method of information sharing as well. It is much easier to misrepresent information in this format. There are no governing agencies for social media to make sure that the information presented is accurate. There are no fact checkers to make sure that agencies are representing information accurately and there is no barrier to prevent hostile or irresponsible responses. This could create a hostile cyber-environment which could easily derail the appropriate conversations.

Whether social media sources have the message correct or not, ASD is being talked about openly and often and that can only contribute to awareness. As a person with ASD or as an advocate for people with ASD it is our responsibility to embrace this coverage and correct the misleading stories when we can. As a strong self-advocate, you can be the one that rights the wrong message shared through social media. While speaking out publicly can be overwhelming and scary, you can speak up through social media. You don't have to speak directly to people, talk in front of a group of people, or worry about the social rules of conversation when advocating in the social media world.

ADVOCATING THROUGH SOCIAL MEDIA

There are many agencies that claim to represent ASD through social media, agencies that claim to be strong advocates, to have the newest ground-breaking therapy, or to have developed the newest technology to "cure" ASD, and these agencies are able to spread their message widely through this channel. The same structure that allows you to become a strong voice for ASD also allows these agencies to spread their message like wildfire. Again, it is up to you to challenge these messages openly. You can do so by posting comments or creating a podcast, a blog, or a Twitter feed that combats the messages globally.

To begin this practice, visit a major social media site and identify a group that claims to represent ASD. Highlight the social media site you choose to investigate from the following group:

Facebook	YouTube	Twitter	Tumblr	Instagram

Once you have chosen the site to investigate, find various postings regarding ASD. Identify and use the lines below to discuss one posting that presents information accurately and one that presents inaccurate information or makes false claims. Once you have identified the post you would like to challenge, develop an appropriate response to submit and share with another advocate:

____

____

____

____

____

____

____

____

____

____

____

____

____

While it isn't necessary to always speak up and be the token ASD person, this action will help society gain a better understanding of what ASD is and how it affects individuals differently. Advocacy is also a difficult thing to manage because it could be very easily turned into a preaching session where people feel like they are being scolded. As with anything it is important to approach advocacy after examining the details and formulating a plan. Advocating is something you have control over. You do not have control over what is being posted, but you can control the education you provide.

There are many positive benefits of social media for making links with others throughout the world. This can be a great avenue for people with ASD to connect with people with shared interests. Where previously, people may have lived lonely lives with very few people to communicate with, the world has become an open line of communication for everyone. This has incredible benefits for developing a sense of place for those who have struggled for so long to feel like they belong anywhere.

SOCIAL MEDIA ADVOCACY PRACTICE

Advocacy is an art that takes practice. If not done in a well-thought-out way, your advocacy could be construed as rude or overbearing. Practice how you could respond through comments on a social media site in the role of an educator and advocate for the ASD community.

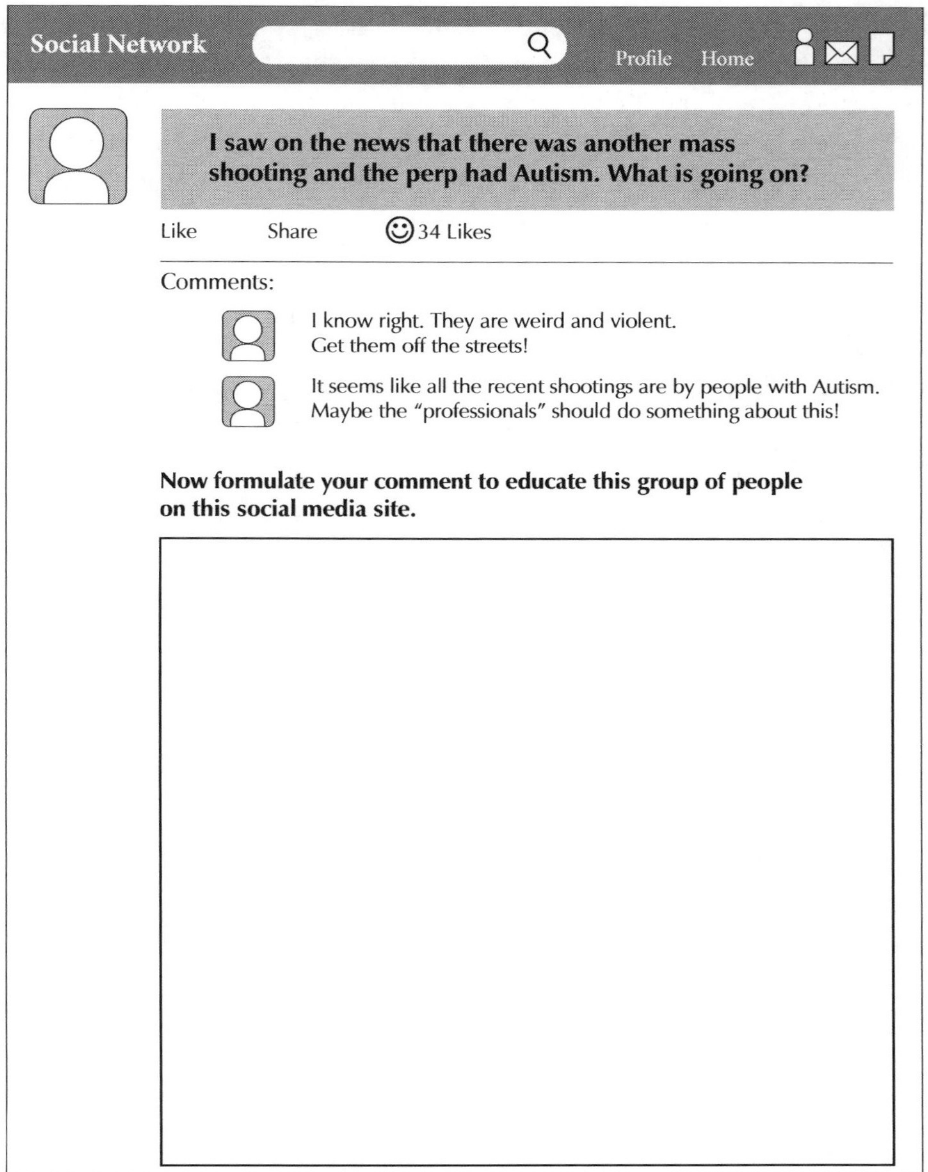

At the conclusion of Chapter 3, we are going to transition our discussion from self-perception to recognizing individual strengths and learning how to use those strengths to reframe your view and to prepare for a career after college. In the first chapter, you explored your personal stories and the impact they have had on your self-perception as you developed into an adult college student. Next, you had the opportunity to recognize how language can be construed to impact a positive or negative self-perception.

Finally, in the third chapter, you worked through the influences of different channels of information demonstrated through the media and their projection on your self-perception, noting that you have a chance through social media to advocate for yourself and others with ASD. To summarize, your efforts up to this point have been focused on a recognition of how external factors, like media and language, and personal stories impact how your self-perception contributes to your worldview.

The next step is to transition your focus from self-perception to learning about and utilizing your strengths, core values, and personality to reframe your view as a young adult with ASD. In the next chapter, you will review some established strengths evident in ASD as you identify your own strengths and use them to reframe negative self-perceptions. Next, you will develop core identity values and examine both the polarity and intersection between your values. You can use that knowledge to understand the purpose of social rules and how to build a strong team. Finally, we will introduce the idea of changing the goal from simply reaching academic and social demands to actively and intentionally preparing for a career. Since you have worked through understanding self-perception, our focus shifts now to the factors that contribute to a full acknowledgment of your identity and how you can project your strengths and values as you interact with the college world around you. Reflect on what you have learned in this chapter and evaluate yourself honestly using the BASICS chart.

BACK TO BASICS

Consider these guiding questions as you prepare to evaluate yourself.

B	**Behavior**	Are you keeping up with current media events? Are you engaging with social media appropriately? Do you advocate for people with ASD through the media? Are you monitoring the trends in media depictions of ASD? What are you doing to maintain a positive perspective of ASD?
A	**Academics**	Are you attending all your classes on time? Are you consistenly using your organizational strategies? What are you saying about your organizational system? Are you keeping up with everything?
S	**Self-care**	Are you getting enough sleep? Are you eating healthily? Are you planning for your self-care activities? Are you keeping your space clean? What are you doing to make sure you are managing your stress level?
I	**Interaction**	Are you checking in with your support team? Are you planning time for social activities? Are you actively engaged in classes? What are you doing to get to know your roommates? Are you checking your email/blackboard daily?
C	**Community**	Do you feel like you belong? Are you asking for help when needed? Have you met anyone new? Do you know the names of any classmates? Are you involved in anything socially?
S	**Self-monitoring**	Are you managing your time? Are you accepting critical feedback? Are you managing your frustration level? Are you willing to see the perspectives of others? Are you advocating for yourself?

BACK TO BASICS: RATE YOURSELF

B	**Behavior** 1 2 3	**Comments**
A	**Academics** 1 2 3	**Comments**
S	**Self-care** 1 2 3	**Comments**
I	**Interaction** 1 2 3	**Comments**
C	**Community** 1 2 3	**Comments**
S	**Self-monitoring** 1 2 3	**Comments**

GOALS

Personal:

Academic:

Social:

Chapter 4

IDENTIFYING YOUR STRENGTHS

Knowing what your gifts are is the first step in sharing your gifts with the world.

INTRODUCTION

The traits that typically go hand in hand with an ASD are largely viewed as negative traits that cause hindrances in the social and emotional development of individuals with the diagnosis. Perhaps a person with ASD is highly focused on the interworking of computer systems or mathematical equations. This focus could be seen as obsessive if viewed negatively, or highly engaged if viewed positively. A person with ASD who is socially quirky and makes attempts to engage people through scripted activities could be seen as insincere but if viewed through a more positive lens, this same person could be seen as a creative and talented actor or comedian. Finally, a person with ASD who would rather work alone to solve problems creatively could be seen as isolative and disengaged if viewed negatively; however, that same person could be the most effective and efficient employee if this trait was viewed more positively.

To stereotype people with ASD as people of genius intellect would be a gross misinterpretation. However, creativity and acts of genius in specific areas are highly likely in this specific population. Genius can be viewed as something original or creative that brings about change. In this view of genius, it is plausible that the original and creative approaches to problem solving, thinking patterns and artistic ability that could go along with a diagnosis of ASD could be seen as genius. Creative and intelligent people with ASD often spend countless hours focused on specific work to discover or create something new—something that could impact people or change the way things are done. Because they are not as attached to the social world and all the implications that go along with that, people with ASD are not so dependent on social approval. Instead, they more often get their self-rewards from the work they do and the discoveries they make. This narrowed focus and intense commitment to their work allows for incredible breakthroughs in many areas. This creative genius is the foundation of the characteristics of ASD. If people with ASD choose the right field of study and career, they have the potential to be incredibly successful.

In a study over a century ago, Iles (1906) identified many characteristics of inventors. Some of these characteristics included analytic ability, originality of thought, perseverance, suspicion, optimism, analysis, competence, observation, and intelligence among others. In that same study, the inventors themselves identified the characteristics as perseverance, imagination, keen observation skills, mechanical ability, and memory. Perhaps the most striking observation about inventors is their ability to work for countless hours on the same project, with failed attempt after failed attempt, and to persevere with patience and focus until the final product is successfully developed. These identified qualities of expert inventors are often present in the personality characteristics of people with ASD.

To further examine the characteristics of leaders in specific fields, the field of mathematics could be identified as another great fit for people with ASD. Mathematicians tend to have many characteristics that are aligned with ASD. Some of these include an intense and narrow area of focus, the ability to see patterns in all things, independent thinking, being analytical in reasoning, systematic thinking, the ability to be content working with numbers instead of people all day, the ability to become consumed with a problem until it is solved, the ability to think of creative solutions to the same problem until a solution is reached, and the perseverance and patience to maintain focus for hours upon hours until the work is finished. Again, these characteristics of expert mathematicians are often observable in people with ASD as well.

Another potential area of great success for people with ASD could be the field of hard sciences. Chemistry, biology, physics, etc. are all fields that value the ability of scientists to focus narrowly with little social interaction for hours, days, or even weeks until a breakthrough is made. The characteristics of genius scientists could include a desire to comprehensively understand the topic studied, logically based thinking, originality, thinking free of biases, the ability to suspend judgment, perseverance and patience. Perhaps the most respected quality of successful scientists is the ability to develop original thought not based on previous experts in the field, but grounded in true curiosity. Again, many of these characteristics are aligned with the personalities of people with ASD.

A field that is often overlooked as a potentially successful field of study/career for people with ASD is the field of liberal arts. Whether it is music, visual arts, or theatre, it is very possible that some of the most successful artists have some identified ASD qualities as well. Some of the qualities necessary to be successful in this field are the ability to see patterns, visual thinking, creativity, fascination with specific objects, intense memory for details, originality, focus, the ability to work in solitude, and, specifically for theatre, the ability to memorize a script and take on a role with specific and identified characteristics. Many people with ASD share these same qualities and due to the primary characteristic of identifying patterns, they often excel in the area of liberal arts.

LESSON 1: SUCCESS AND ASD QUALITIES

To better identify the ASD characteristics in specific people who have been viewed as geniuses in their respective fields, we will now present a description of some well-known people and readers can identify the traits of ASD that may be present within the description.

ISAAC NEWTON

Isaac Newton is a very well-known physicist and mathematician. He is often referred to as an enigmatic genius (Fitzgerald and O'Brien 2007) and there is no denying that his life's work had a substantial impact on his field. He is described as being very grounded in logic and a strict rule follower. He was impacted at an early age by the specifics of mathematics and mechanical workings, often reading and studying for hours on end with no breaks for eating or sleeping. Although Isaac Newton did poorly in school, he was an autodidact. Through his intense focus, he taught himself advanced mathematics in just a few years.

Socially, Isaac Newton has been described as withdrawn and isolated by his work. Newton revered his work over people and could become so distracted by his work that he was considered a loner. It is difficult to find evidence of relationships in biographies about Isaac Newton. While there are a few accounts of romantic relationships, those did not last long and there is very little evidence present of solid friendships outside of working partners.

Newton was a strict record keeper with all things in his life. He exhibited control through detailed accounts of financial records, diary entries, experiment notes, and lab reports. He often attempted to control the people around him by forcing them to focus on his narrow interest areas. He set many rules for his life and expected those around him to comply with his rules as well. This often made him appear arrogant and egocentric.

What characteristics used to describe Isaac Newton could be aligned with ASD?

____

____

____

____

____

____

____

____

____

____

NIKOLA TESLA

Nikola Tesla was a brilliant inventor and engineer. In fact, he is a favorite of many contemporary engineers today. He is regarded as being more gifted than the better-known inventor, Thomas Edison, who reportedly exploited Tesla (Fitzgerald and O'Brien 2007) and claimed many of his ideas as his own without Tesla even knowing it was happening. Although many inventors and engineers of that time had odd social and work habits, Tesla was considered far more eccentric than most others. He is described as a reclusive workaholic who had many distinct phobias and obsessions. One of these obsessions was with the number three. Tesla only stayed in hotel rooms with numbers that were divisible by three, he walked around the block three times before entering the building and he required 18 napkins, also divisible by three, to polish his silver and glassware each night.

Nikola Tesla worked very hard and often would not stop working until a project or invention was completed. It was not outside the norm for him to work until 3:00 am, sleep for two hours then wake up and work again. It is reported (Fitzgerald and O'Brien 2007) that he once worked for 84 hours straight without rest. While he did not get a full night's sleep, Tesla did admit to dozing off occasionally.

Socially, Tesla was a recluse. Although he did have a few close friends, he preferred working in solitude rather than attending social events and participating in chitchat. He came across as arrogant and egocentric with others and often had difficulties maintaining relationships. He also chose to live a life of celibacy and did not engage in romantic relationships at any time. Later in life, Tesla developed a fondness for pigeons and would spend time feeding them and talking with them as if they were friends.

Nikola Tesla was most known for having a photographic memory. Once he visualized something, he was able to remember every detail about the object. In addition, he visualized all of his inventions and saw them in working order in his mind. He was able to discuss these detailed visualizations but never developed a drawing of them on paper.

Finally, Nikola Tesla had many phobias and sensitivities. Among these were intense sensitivities to sound and light. He often controlled his physical environment to avoid the impact of these sensitivities. In addition, he could not touch hair or shake hands with people. He was against any kind of jewelry and that apparent aversion to jewelry developed into an aversion specifically to pearls, which developed further into an intense disgust for all round objects.

What characteristics used to describe Nikola Tesla could be aligned with ASD?

____

____

____

____

____

____

____

DAN AYKROYD

Dan Aykroyd is a gifted comedian, actor, screenwriter and singer. He is most known for his roles on *Saturday Night Live* where he was a talented comedian. In addition, his roles in *Ghostbusters* and *The Blues Brothers* are staples of pop culture from the 1980s.

As a child, Dan Aykroyd had many symptoms that made him socially nervous. He had verbal and physical tics that caused him to be anxious around others. He also had obsessions with both ghosts and law enforcement (Miller 2013). These intense interests were considered odd for his age, but they continue to this day and he continues to carry a police badge. These intense areas of interests and lifelong studying of ghosts and law enforcement contributed to the writing of the screenplays for both *Ghostbusters* and *The Blues Brothers*.

Aykroyd was considered eccentric and a hard worker, often spending sleepless nights writing screenplays and creating new characters. In addition, he is very detailed in business planning and reporting and has successfully started and continues to maintain several businesses.

What characteristics used to describe Dan Aykroyd could be aligned with ASD?

____

____

____

____

____

____

____

____

____

____

____

DARYL HANNAH

Daryl Hannah is a talented and noted A-list actress who starred in such movies as *Splash*, *Kill Bill*, and *Wall Street*. As a teen, she followed her love of film and moved from her family home in Chicago to Los Angeles at the age of 17 to pursue an acting career. In addition, Daryl Hannah is an environmental activist who lives off the grid and has been arrested several times for standing up for her beliefs.

As a child, Daryl Hannah was painfully shy and would frequently rock herself to soothe her anxiety (Cooper 2013). She was isolated in school and frequently would tune the teacher out and miss important information. Doctors told her mother that she would need to be medicated and institutionalized for her behaviors, but her mother refused.

During her pre-teen years, Daryl Hannah turned to movies as her escape. She has been quoted as saying that movies and acting were her "Oz" allowing her to escape from her tormented reality. She would spend hours watching old movies and studying the acting qualities within each film. Although she was still intensely shy and detested being the center of attention, this affinity for film encouraged her acting pursuit.

As an adult, the continued fear of social situations caused her to leave the Hollywood scene. She was noticeably absent from the premieres of her own movies, she refused to do any promotional activities on talk shows, and would rarely attend award ceremonies. She still acts occasionally but her passion is living an eco-friendly life and she continues to be an activist for her environmental protection beliefs.

What characteristics used to describe Daryl Hannah could be aligned with ASD?

____

____

____

____

____

____

____

____

____

____

____

____

LESSON 2: IDENTIFYING THE ESTABLISHED STRENGTHS IN ASD

As you work through this chapter, our goal is to encourage you to not only recognize your individual strengths as a person with ASD, but also to reframe negative perceptions into positive ones. This idea of reframing your view takes some conscious practice, but it is important that you can see yourself positively and project confidence in a social world. Your ideas, thoughts, attitudes, and actions are unique and worth offering, especially as you start engaging in college social life and casual networking. Confidence in yourself and your strengths in spite of any negative stereotypes or attitudes about ASD in the media or your personal stories helps you to portray a positive and meaningful image that reflects your identity. A good place to start reflecting on your strengths is to think about those that are already contributed to people who are on the autism spectrum.

We have discussed some of the characteristics that icons such as Isaac Newton and Dan Aykroyd possess and how those characteristics are displayed through their work. Newton's record keeping and attention to detail, commonly associated with ASD, were certainly strengths when it came to his logic-based work. Aykroyd utilized a unique special interest in ghosts to his benefit in what is perhaps his most famous role in the movie *Ghostbusters*. These uniquely "Aspie" characteristics are strengths when we consider their incredible impact. Here is a list of some commonly recognized strengths associated with people with ASD. People who have autism:

- have a fascination for details and facts
- are especially sensitive to the external sensory environment, allowing for a unique experience with the environment
- have excellent overall memory
- can retain focus on topics of interest for a long time
- have an ability to intensely analyze information that is of interest
- are loyal, honest, and dependable
- are literal thinkers
- desire routine and accuracy.

These strengths associated with ASD have changed the world. The most creative and innovative brains push society forward and people with autism certainly have unique brains. People who are extremely passionate and persevere are successful more often than people are successful by chance. The more deeply one knows about any one thing, or any one intense interest, the more impact this person can have when their energies are exerted concerning it. Rigid adherence to a schedule makes for a dependable employee. People with ASD can look for common strengths that are associated with unique brains and experiences, finding refreshingly positive perceptions.

You might consider what perceptions people have of you in order to see what strengths are noted that are also attributed to those established strengths often associated with students with ASD. The group of words shown in Figure 4.1 is a representation of the most commonly used words, known as a "wordle," used by the families, friends, and instructors of a group of college students with autism. The words that appear the largest are those used most often. For example, you can see that the words "honest" and "loyal" are larger, which represents the repetition of those words in other people's descriptions of this group of students with autism.

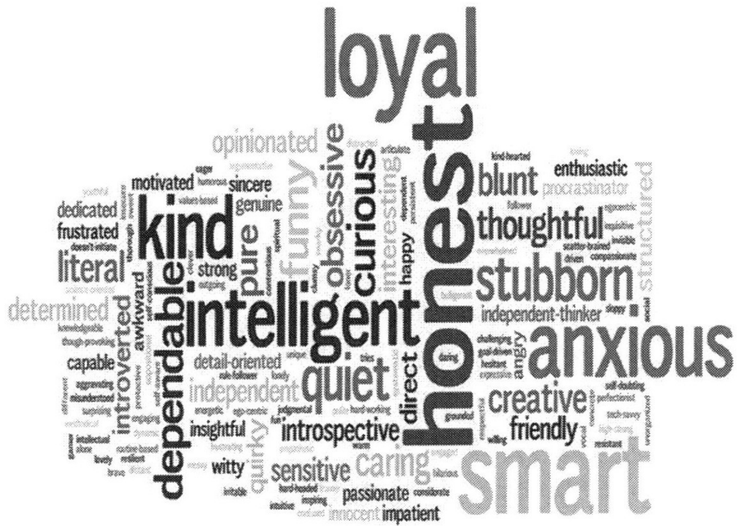

FIGURE 4.1: ADVOCATE PERCEPTIONS

In this next activity, you will have a chance to create your own visual representation of the words people use to describe you. Follow the directions in order to develop your own graphic image of the perception that people have of you.

CREATING A VISUAL REPRESENTATION OF PERCEPTIONS OF ASD

- Step 1: Ask several family members, friends, mentors, and/or teachers to write down as many words as they can think of that describe you as someone who has ASD. Collect their lists.
- Step 2: Tally each word as it occurs in the various lists you have collected. Each word should have a tally of the number of times it occurred on the lists. For example, "intelligent" might appear five times, while "kind" might appear six times.
- Step 3: Rank the words by the tallies, from highest to lowest.
- Step 4: Create your own visual representation that looks similar to the one in this book. To do that, you can use size and any other signifier you want, like color, to demonstrate which words people associate with you. You can use the space below to compile and tally your words. There are a few boxes that you can use to help you get started. Write the word that occurs most frequently in the largest box, the second word that appears most frequently in the next largest box, and so on. Words that occurred fewer times will be written smaller.

HOW OTHERS VIEW YOU AS A PERSON WITH ASD

LESSON 3: RECOGNIZING YOUR INDIVIDUAL STRENGTHS

You can use the positive characteristics that others use to describe you to help you get started with thinking about what you identify as your strengths. Sometimes other perspectives can give you real insight to an aspect of yourself you had not considered until it has been pointed out to you. Others might recognize your strengths before you think of them as strengths. Other times, your own interests and your work are your strengths that you are not only aware of, but also actively work on to sharpen their effectiveness.

Let us start by thinking about the most often used words others used to describe you as someone who has ASD. Refer to the previous activity and the words you collected from people who know you. Then, you can think about whether or not you agree that this is a strength you feel you have. If we were to do this with our example "wordle" that represents a group of college students as perceived by their family members, friends, and instructors, these words would be their Top Five. We have italicized some words that the students individually identified as their strengths.

1. *Honest*
2. Smart
3. Loyal
4. *Intelligent*
5. Kind

Write down your Top Five words and circle the words that you think are some of your strengths:

1. ____
2. ____
3. ____
4. ____
5. ____

What strengths do you see in yourself that are not listed in those that others pointed out in you?

There are many ways to think about what your strengths are. You might consider the kind of work you do and whether or not you are effective at it. This, for many college students, might be a strength associated with a particular academic subject or unique skill. It will also help to think about the individual steps at work in your interactions with others, your academic work, how you present yourself in the classroom, and other experiences. Think about whether you are a strong logical thinker or if you excel at thinking in a unique visual way. Consider whether you are a skilled musician because you have natural talent or because you can demonstrate perseverance to engage in the repetitive practice involved in the mastery of an instrument. In other words, what is it, exactly, that you do very well? Perhaps you can understand contemporary physics theories and explain them very simply to others. Maybe you can name the country associated with any flag at your first glance at it. Start with what you know you are interested in and see how your interest plays out in your life. This is likely to be a strength you have and recognizing it can be a very effective catalyst in your pursuit of career and personal interests. Seeing your strengths as they are demonstrated through a special interest serves to solidify your interest and ability to pursue it.

LESSON 4: REPLACING NEGATIVE SELF-PERCEPTIONS

We all have pieces of our personality that could be viewed as negative by ourselves or other people. It is important to remember that each piece of your personality makes a difference in how you are perceived and how you perceive yourself, and some aspects perceived negatively might actually be quite positive if you practice replacing negative self-perceptions with positive benefits. It is important to remember it could be true that not every trait you have has a positive benefit. But, identifying which traits are truly negative and have negative impacts on your life or others' lives is the first step to working out a plan to make sure you work to improve in whatever area it is.

You have worked through quite a few discussions of identity and recognizing your strengths in this text so far. In order to approach the process of replacing negative perceptions you have of yourself, you need to take a moment to write down those negative perceptions so that you can then work on replacing them with more positive perceptions. You cannot replace negative self-talk with positive benefits if you have not sorted out what negative self-talk looks like for you. Self-talk is what you think about yourself and tell yourself. For example, perhaps you react poorly to a change in the location of your group project meeting and think to yourself, "I really hate when things change but when I act upset and am too rigid, I feel like everyone in my group gets annoyed with me." You can use a log to write down the times that you experience negative self-talk.

SELF-TALK LOG

Use this page to log your own negative self-talk for at least one day. Write what you thought on the left and what triggered those thoughts on the right. Then, in the next exercise, you can use the negative self-talk points you wrote down to practice replacing negative self-perceptions with positive benefits.

Negative self-talk:	**Trigger:**
Example: "Being rigid annoys my group"	I was upset and rude when the group meeting location changed

REPLACING NEGATIVE SELF-PERCEPTIONS PRACTICE

To practice replacing negative self-talk with positive benefits, you can use a table that provides space for the personal traits you pointed out under "Negative self-talk" in your self-talk log, and then think of how that trait might also be a positive benefit for you. We have listed four traits and positive benefits to help you get started. If you are having trouble thinking of a positive benefit, you might discuss that particular trait with someone else to see if his or her perspective is a positive one.

Trait	**Positive benefit**
Guarded	Keeps individuals from getting hurt
Naïve	Allows individuals to maintain a positive outlook on life
Blunt	Keeps the individual from being misunderstood
Rigid	People will always know what to expect

LESSON 5: REFRAMING YOUR VIEW

When you practice reframing your view, allowing for a truly positive perception, you can filter out negative perceptions that prevent you from trying something new, thinking in an unconventional way, or simply from feeling the best you can feel about yourself. Knowing what you do well and what interests you and how those two elements are connected is an important step that many people learn as college students. College is generally an environment that fosters independence and the development of identity through experience and choice. It is, in many ways, a prime context for you to practice reframing your view.

College is meant to be a platform for identifying strengths and using them. After all, for many college students with the goal of post-graduation employment, you will need to have a firm grasp on what you are good at and why someone should hire you. Reframing using the college context to guide your practice can help you situate yourself within the process of reframing your view.

Think about one of the traits that you identified in the table from your negative self-talk log. You will complete the following exercise thinking only about that trait and how it impacts you on the college campus. In the column on the left, write about how the particular trait might present itself in any of the settings listed. For example, if you are rigid and not flexible, this might impact you during a presentation if the classroom computer does not work when you had been counting on using your PowerPoint slides. To reframe that rigid thinking in the presentation setting, you might be so determined to use your PowerPoint slides that you think to use your laptop to open the file and show your slides. Remember, though, that not all traits will necessarily be positive in a given setting. For example, being especially rigid at a party is the opposite of what people expect when they are trying to relax and have a good time. Use the following table to practice reframing one of your own traits in various elements of the college setting.

TRAIT:

SETTING	REFRAMING
Food court:	
Classroom:	
Lab project:	
Party:	

When you work to focus on positive perceptions, you will nurture your strengths and see increasingly how they are associated with the characteristics of ASD. As you read in Chapter 2, the language you associate with and use can impact not only how other people perceive you, but also how you view yourself. Combining what you know about identity language and recognizing your strengths, you can navigate college and the years after with more confidence. Identifying your strengths helps you put your skills and talents to use and to learn in a meaningful way those skills that you need to develop as you take your next steps in internships and careers.

There are many strengths associated with ASD that you might have always possessed only to learn in college how to reframe them as positive characteristics or benefits that can significantly impact how you see yourself. Learning about those characteristics of ASD that are positive and suggest a unique and valuable way of understanding the world can help you identify some of the qualities that you can identify with and recognize as a strength. For example, considering some of the characteristics of Nikola Tesla and how they are associated with ASD, you might begin to understand eccentric qualities as positive attributes when they lead to unique and interesting discoveries or skills, like Tesla's desire to skip sleep in order to work. You might not associate yourself with all of the characteristics of ASD, but you can learn to think positively about those with which you do associate. Knowing what your strengths are makes the process of reframing your view much easier. Start with your strengths and see how they impact your attitudes, actions, and perceptions. You might see patterns emerge that can lead you to meaningful relationships, careers, classes, or situations that emphasize your interests. After all, enjoying what you do is easier when you know it utilizes your strengths.

Take some time to reflect on the difficult work you have done in this chapter. It is never easy to try to change how you view yourself and shift your outlook that has been with you for years. Use the BASICS chart to honestly evaluate yourself on the work you completed in this chapter.

BACK TO BASICS

Consider these guiding questions as you prepare to evaluate yourself.

B	**Behavior**	Have you identified your strengths? Are you connecting with established strengths of ASD? Are you monitoring negative self-talk? Do you actively practice reframing your view? Are your strengths evident in your behavior?
A	**Academics**	Are you attending all your classes on time? Are you applying organizational strategies? Are you consistently using your organizational system? Are you keeping up with everything?
S	**Self-care**	Are you getting enough sleep? Are you eating healthily? Are you planning for your self-care activities? Are you keeping your space clean? What are you doing to make sure you are managing your stress level?
I	**Interaction**	Are you checking in with your support team? Are you planning time for social activities? Are you actively engaged in classes? What are you doing to get to know your roommates? Are you checking your email/blackboard daily?
C	**Community**	Do you feel like you belong? Are you asking for help when needed? Have you met anyone new? Do you know the names of any classmates? Are you involved in anything socially?
S	**Self-monitoring**	Are you managing your time? Are you accepting critical feedback? Are you managing your frustration level? Are you willing to see the perspectives of others? Are you advocating for yourself?

BACK TO BASICS: RATE YOURSELF

B	**Behavior** 1 2 3	**Comments**
A	**Academics** 1 2 3	**Comments**
S	**Self-care** 1 2 3	**Comments**
I	**Interaction** 1 2 3	**Comments**
C	**Community** **1 2 3**	**Comments**
S	**Self-monitoring** 1 2 3	**Comments**

GOALS

Personal:

Academic:

Social:

Chapter 5

DEVELOPING YOUR CORE IDENTITY

Your thoughts, feelings, and beliefs are your foundation.

INTRODUCTION

Core identity can be described as the foundation or the building blocks for what makes up a person and defines them at their core. These are the values that a person adheres to when making any decision, the feelings that guide their reactions to situations, and the belief system that helps give a person direction and purpose in his or her life. These values could have been introduced during childhood by parents and grandparents or taught by an influential teacher in elementary school. These values, also described as core identity features, could also be tied to positive life experiences such as having a solid family upbringing during developmental years. If these core identity features are tied to positive life experiences, they typically mirror those values of the influential people. These values could also be tied to negative life experiences such as bullying or feeling isolated. If these core identity features are tied to those negative life experiences, they are typically the driving force to make things better for other people.

Throughout the beginning of this text, discussions have been focused on defining how previous experiences have been integral in the development of perceptions of ASD and the ability to value the strengths associated with an autism spectrum diagnosis. This information has been offered to help readers develop insight into how their own worldview has developed. This insight is vital because all of these life experiences, both positive and negative, play a significant role in shaping who a person is, how that person develops self-worth, how that person develops his or her core identity, and how that person interacts with others.

From this point forward, readers will have the opportunity to challenge their previous core identity features and solidify the features with which they still identify. Experiences during this time in life help people make decisions about who they are and what they stand for as they grow into adulthood. While it is incredibly important to know identity foundation and how values develop, it is also acceptable to challenge those historical views on life and adjust according to new views. People see life through different lenses depending on what they learn from various encounters with people from diverse backgrounds and belief systems. This opportunity for growth is what allows people to develop core identity with purpose rather than simply inheriting a belief system.

One notable strength related to people with ASD is the ability to stay true to their core identity once it is developed with purpose. Once a person with ASD develops these values and beliefs, that person typically is not easily persuaded by peers to go against those established guiding principles. Individuals with ASD usually fully commit to these values as reliable guiding factors to make life's decisions, but because they are so steadfast in the commitment to these values, people with ASD sometimes struggle with allowing their values to shift as social norms evolve.

Developing a strong understanding of core identity is vital at this stage in life. Students will work to distinguish what they believe in from what others have taught them, and it will help them develop true identity while helping to grow strong personal and professional boundaries. Young adults occasionally struggle with this process because they relate their commitment to these established core values as an equal commitment to the person who taught them these values. A shift in core identity systems does not equate to a betrayal of those who taught the values initially nor does it mean that a person with ASD is challenged to change who they are as a person. The challenge is to embrace identified core identity features while also recognizing the impact those features may have on others. Developing these core identity features in a studious way, taking into account the impact on others, is necessary to make the established values work in the context of your life socially. Individuals with ASD typically construct their identities through their core values, whereas neurotypical individuals more often have socially constructed identities. By strategically implementing core values into the social rules, which will be discussed in detail in later in the next chapter, a person with ASD can create his or her own social context. When that occurs it is likely that a community of like-minded individuals will be identified and a sense of place can be established.

Throughout this chapter students will work through activities that will provoke thought and will help develop an understanding of core identity and its features. Students will also explore why these features are important to personal foundation, how they work into social norms, and how the intersection makes them unique as individuals. The most important thing to remember during this process is that each person defines core identity differently and there is no right or wrong answer to what is important.

LESSON 1: IDENTIFYING WHAT MAKES YOU CALM, PASSIONATE, AND ANXIOUS

One of the first steps in establishing what makes up your core identity is deciphering what drives you emotionally. Identifying the topics that make you calm, passionate, and those things that make you anxious can help you gain insight into the values that have meaning to you at your core. These established values that develop your core identity also dictate how you interact with others. Every person has their own set of core identity features that are driven by values. It is your responsibility to recognize the values that you subscribe to while also respecting the core values that drive other people. Every person has values they can discuss frequently and tirelessly, but they can do so without emotion. An example of values that do not typically draw a charged emotional reaction is honesty. While people would like to live honestly, they are not often emotionally charged over supporting this way of life. People with ASD often choose to live honestly, but do not engage in debates, or arguments over how to encourage honesty in others. This would be a value that encourages a calm state and allows for reflective decision making. Contemplate the values you subscribe to that allow you to engage calmly with others.

Identify five values that you believe in that also make you calm:

1. ______________________________
2. ______________________________
3. ______________________________
4. ______________________________
5. ______________________________

It is also very important to recognize the core values that give you a positive emotional charge. These values typically are matters that you are very enthusiastic about and include values that you could discuss at length without being derailed. These core values are typically the cause of many lengthy discussions due to the unwavering commitment and passion associated with the subject matter. Passion often drives commitment, so it is difficult to inhibit the emotional charge that accompanies these core values. These values are often the subjects that give you energy and guide the decision making. An example of a core value that makes people with ASD passionate is the idea of social justice. This core value passionately encourages people to become strong advocates for marginalized populations. Whether people choose to advocate for others because they have been treated very well by others regardless of differences, or if the passionate feeling is developed out of a need to educate others so people are not treated poorly, the passion is the same. If a value is one that drives a passionate emotional response, it will typically be a primary core identity feature that will not be easily altered.

Identify five values that you believe in that also make you passionate:

1. ______________________________
2. ______________________________
3. ______________________________
4. ______________________________
5. ______________________________

Finally, it is imperative to recognize the values you hold that cause a negative charge to you or others. While these values may be instilled at a very young age and you may faithfully commit to these values, others may not endorse the same values. This does not remove the significance this value contributes to your core identity. However, if this value elicits an anxious reaction from others, it could, in turn, create anxiety for you in social situations. These core values are often the subject of many arguments and social miscues due to the emotions associated with the subject matter. These values are often associated with religion, politics, or sexual orientation and can often be identified as the "no-go" topics of conversation with many people. Again, these values are no less important to your core identity, but it is necessary to recognize and temper your reactions to others to avoid offending others while defending your values.

Identify five values that you believe in that also make you or others anxious:

1. ______________________________
2. ______________________________
3. ______________________________
4. ______________________________
5. ______________________________

As you begin your work to develop your true core identity, keep in mind that the existence of these values within your core identity is not a permit to offend others. Other people also have values and core identity features that carry the same importance to them. It is necessary to take the perspective of others into account during any social interaction and recognize that each person is also working to define his or her own core identity with values that are just as important to them as your values are to you. It is not your role to try to persuade another person to subscribe to your same belief system, nor is it your responsibility to adjust your core identity to be accepted by others. It is your responsibility, though, to respect the values that others commit to with the same level of respect you expect from them.

Identify three core values from each area that may contribute to the make-up of your core identity:

Calm	Passionate	Anxious

Reflect on what makes these values important enough to you to carry them over in your development of your core identity. You may need to defend these values as people try to pressure you to make decisions that are not aligned with them. Circle the top five values that mean the most to you and, using the space below, clarify why they are important.

LESSON 2: DEVELOPING YOUR CORE IDENTITY FEATURES

After you have explored the values that make you calm, passionate, and anxious, the next step in this process is to develop an understanding of how this information can help you identify your core identity features. The values that you discussed in the previous lesson can lend some important perspective on what you truly value at your core. The values that you carry with you that may make you passionate are typically the values that make up part of your core foundation. These values drive us to work hard and make contributions that may foster growth in those value areas. For example, if social justice is a value that makes you passionate, this value may translate into being one of the core identity features that make up your foundation as a person who seeks opportunities to help others. Conversely, a value that you approach in a calm state with very little emotional energy attached may be a value that has some importance to you, but may not be high enough on the level of importance to include it as a core value. Finally, if you have identified a value that is very important to you but you know that it causes you or others with whom you interact anxiety, this value can also be included in the group of values that make up your core identity, but you may want to identify the negative charge that could accompany this feature so you can become self-monitoring in your interactions with people.

The features that make up our core identity serve as directions for how we make decisions. Your core identity features must be nurtured and respected and developed as you enter into adulthood. You will be faced with many difficult decisions and will have your values challenged, but respecting this core identity system will help you remain consistent and make responsible decisions. By appreciating how core identity features impact decision making, you can become mature and responsible in this process. To further analyze the impact of core identity features on our daily lives, they can be separated into three main areas. These areas are defined as thoughts, feelings, and actions.

- *Thoughts*: Core identity features that guide how you view situations and make decisions. The values that fall into this area can help you develop into a mature decision maker who stands strongly aligned with his or her core identity. If you commit to these values, it will be difficult to persuade you to make decisions that do not directly align with your core identity. These core identity features can include things such as being objective, rational, detail oriented, or a seeker of truth.

- *Feelings*: Core identity features that guide your feelings about situations or people. The values that fall into this area can help you approach social interactions with a firm grasp on emotional objectivity. If you commit to these values, you will engage with people in ways that are aligned with your core identity. It will be difficult to persuade you to treat people in ways that do not directly align with these values. These core identity features can include things such as being forgiving, non-judgmental, non-discriminatory, or having a strong sense of justice.

- *Actions*: Core identity features that guide your behaviors and reactions to others. The values that fall into this area can help guide you through social exchanges and the development of relationships. If you commit to these values you will be able to develop and maintain solid relationships with people who have similar values and interests. These features can include being honest, knowing personal limits, being direct, and having a strong work ethic.

To help identify which area your core identity features exist within, examine the previous descriptions and outline on the image below where the core identity features are placed. If the value guides your thoughts, write it on the head. If the value guides your feelings, write it on the heart. If the value guides your actions, write it on the arms and legs.

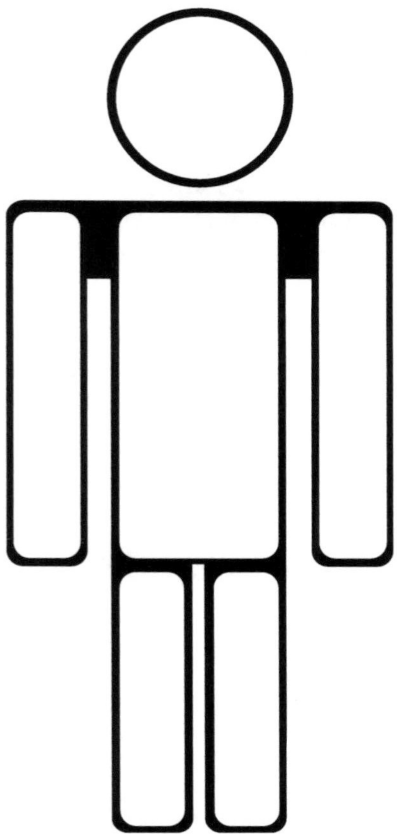

FIGURE 5.1: CORE IDENTITY FEATURES

Consider whether all three areas are represented equally. Are your core identity features more focused in one area than another? If so, your core identity may be skewed and you may need to consider adjusting to ensure that all three areas are represented. This equal representation of values can help you develop into a well-balanced, values-driven person.

Now that you have had the opportunity to work through the process of defining your core identity features in a purposeful way, you should have a set of five, well-balanced and meaningful value statements that will have a positive impact on the development of your core identity. Recognize that these values may shift and change over time as you are challenged by different views; however, your overall core foundation will remain constant.

The final step in your core identity development is to recognize that while the values that make up your core identity are important to your foundation as a person, it is possible to take these values to excess. Any value that makes up your core identity can have a positive or negative effect on others depending on how these values are displayed. If a value is taken to excess, it is possible that relationship development could be stunted and you could offend someone who does not subscribe to the same value.

For each of the five values that you have identified as core identity features, consider the positive and negative impact. For each value, identity the positive impact on your life and relationships as well as the potential negative impact if the values are taken to excess. Use the following diagram to define the potential impact one of these values could have on you and others if not managed responsibly. Choose one of the five values you have identified as your core identity features and write it in the middle star of the blank diagram opposite (Figure 5.3). Carefully consider the positive impact this value could have on you and those around you and document those in the circles. Reflect on how this value could have a negative impact on yourself or others and document those in the rectangles. Being cognizant of the impact of these values as they make up your foundation can be a helpful tool in managing relationships in the social, school, and work setting.

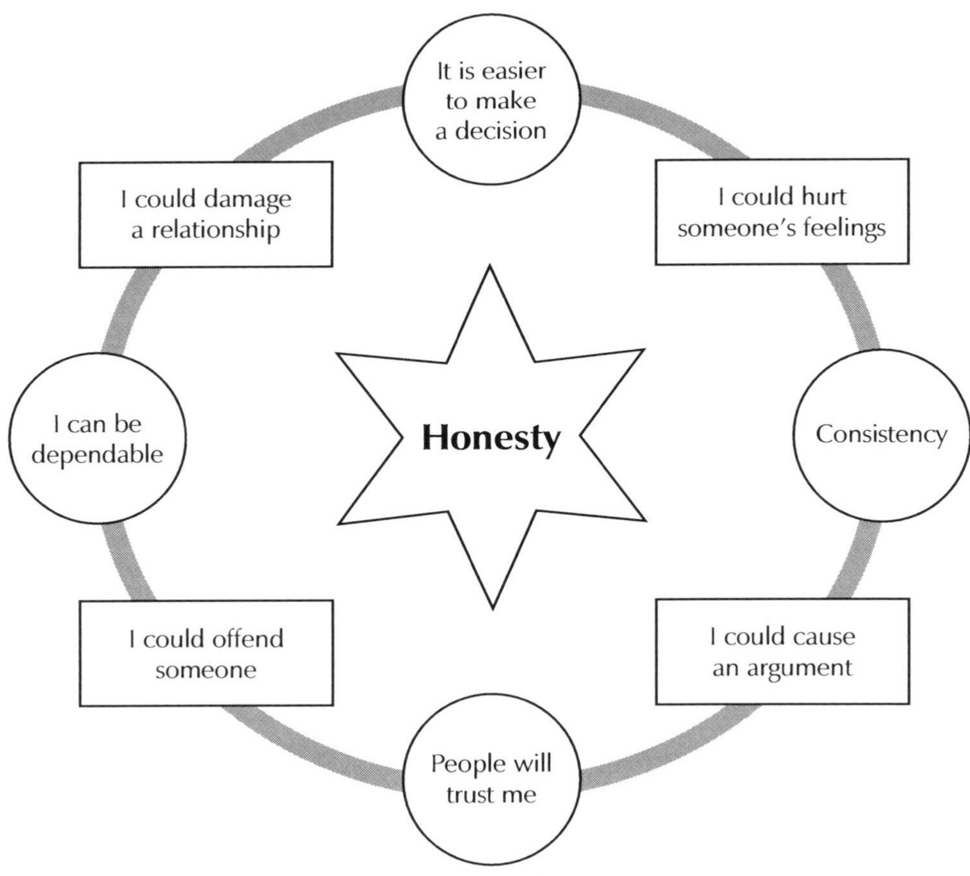

FIGURE 5.2: CORE IDENTITY MODEL (EXAMPLE)

Now use your own values to develop your Core Identity Model.

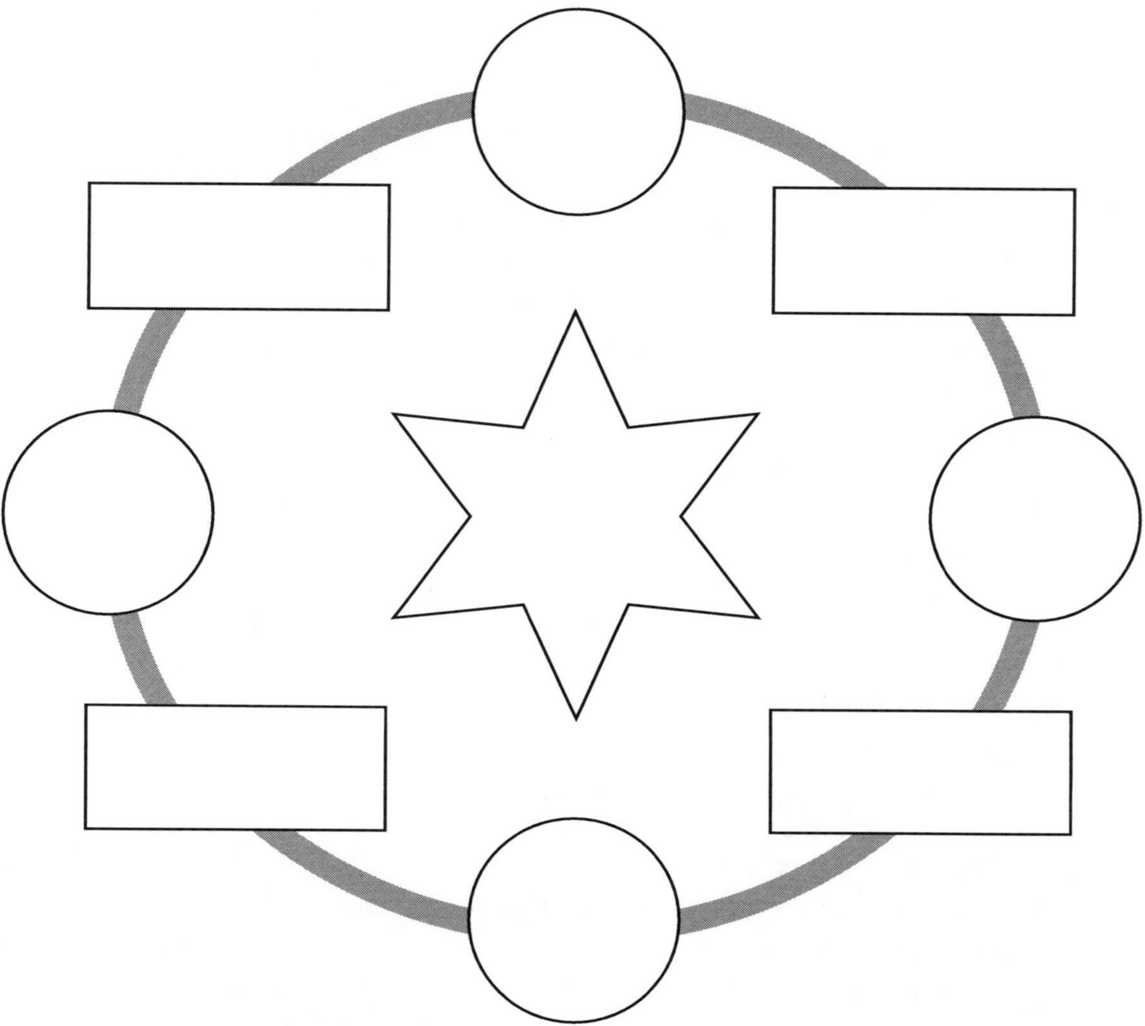

FIGURE 5.3: CORE IDENTITY MODEL

LESSON 3: IT IS RARELY BLACK AND WHITE

People with ASD tend to have magnificent minds full of absolutes, with thinking patterns that are concrete and unwavering, commitment to details that are consistent and predictable, and decisions that are value-driven. This absolute style of thinking can be described as rigid, but it is preferable to view this style of thinking as black-and-white thinking. In this black-and-white style of thinking, people view things as either good or bad, the truth or a lie, people either love you or don't like you. This is often referred to as having a one-track mind (Attwood 1998). Unfortunately, there are very few things in life that are "either/or." As you define your core identity, it is very important to keep in mind that not all things will fall neatly into one definitive category.

The rigid adherence to established values discussed previously can cause anxiety in people with ASD. All circumstances in life are situational and should be approached with an individualized line of thinking. If you cling rigidly to your established values outlined in your core identity without regard to the situation or the inherent nuances, you may experience stress and difficulties when it comes to making hard life decisions, and question your core identity. The stress related to this line of thinking is not necessarily the result of the identified values within your core identity, but is rather a result of black-and-white thinking. Each one of your core identity features inevitably has some flexibility. We call this necessary flexibility the gray area. Much like stress put on a stretching rubber band just before it breaks, the inability to see the shades of gray in any situation can have a negative impact on your social interactions.

Take for example the value of honesty that we have discussed previously. If you rigidly adhere to this value, you may not see the negative impact of responding with rigid honesty until the situation results in a damaged relationship. If a friend asked you to come over for dinner and you do not like the way he cooks, this rigid adherence could cause you to respond by saying, "I don't like the way you cook, so I don't want to come over." This response could hurt your friend's feelings and cause him not to invite you over for any event in the future. Instead of being completely honest in this situation, it would be more appropriate to recognize the gray area and respond by saying, "I would like to come over, but I can't make it to dinner. Let's meet up later." This response is not completely honest and not completely dishonest, but somewhere in the middle.

Develop a brief scenario that may require you to recognize the necessary flexibility in the gray area.

____

____

____

____

What difficulties could surface if you respond according to the black-and-white style of thinking?

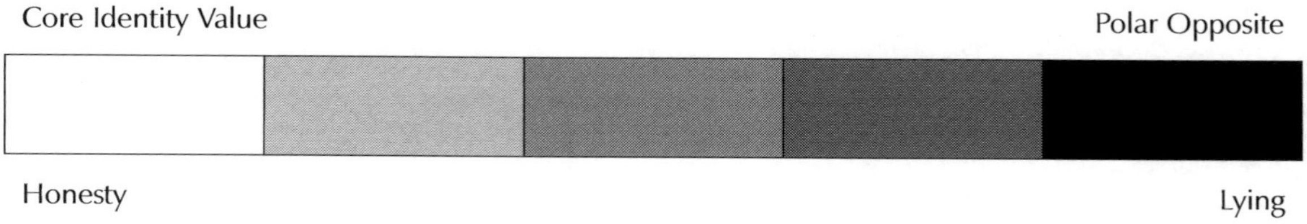

Core Identity Value				Polar Opposite
Honesty				Lying

Gray Area 1: A group asks you to join them for lunch at the cafeteria…

Gray Area 2: Your friend asks you if she looks fat in her new pants…

Gray Area 3: Your mom tells you that she has written a check without money in the account until payday (two days later)…

FIGURE 5.4: IT'S NOT ALWAYS BLACK AND WHITE (EXAMPLE)

Figure 5.4 shows honesty as an example of a core identity value. Potential situations that may fall in the other gray areas in between are identified below the figure.

Consider the values you have identified as features of your core identity. For the purpose of this activity, define your core identity value in the white section and define the polar opposite of that value in the black section of Figure 5.5. Identify potential situations that may fall in the other gray areas in between and the consequences associated with black-and-white thinking.

Core Identity Value				Polar Opposite
________				________

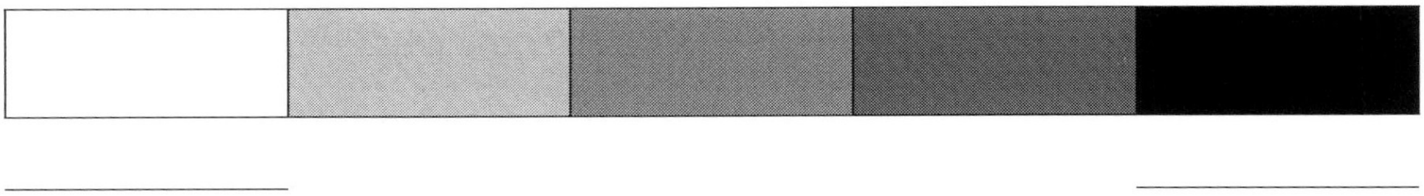

Gray Area 1: ____________________

Gray Area 2: ____________________

Gray Area 3: ____________________

FIGURE 5.5: IT'S NOT ALWAYS BLACK AND WHITE

LESSON 4: THE INTERSECTION OF YOUR CORE IDENTITY FEATURES

As you continue the important work of developing the foundation of your core identity, another idea to keep in mind is the possibility that your core values may intersect awkwardly with each other if you endorse the black-and-white approach to core values. If a person with ASD does not recognize the gray area of situations and allows him or herself to display excesses in those values, confusion and anxiety can erupt. When one value is held too rigidly, the impact may mean breaching another core value.

Take for example, if you hold the value of justice as a primary feature of your core identity and you adhere to the black-and-white thinking, you will see only the laws that are in place to guide our society in a civilized way. If taken to the excess, you may be identified as the gatekeeper of the rules and laws without regard to how people may be impacted by those laws. Consider if another value that makes up your core identity is to never hurt another living thing. Again, if you adhere to the black-and-white thinking, there would be no situation where it would ever make sense to harm someone. These two values could intersect in this unmanageable way.

SCENARIO

You are grocery shopping with your family and notice a young woman with a toddler holding her hand shopping in the aisle next to you. She has a cart with a small number of items in it, but you notice that as she is walking down the aisle, she places two cans of vegetables and a jar of apple sauce in her large purse. You make eye contact with her and she has tears in her eyes. You approach her and tell her that it is against the law to steal and you will need to let the store manager know what you saw. She begins crying and begs you not to tell the manager. She goes on to tell you that she is only taking what is necessary to feed her young child. She explains that her husband has recently passed away and she only has a part-time job with just enough money to pay rent. If you report her to the manager, it is likely she will be arrested and lose her child as well.

How have your core values intersected in this one scenario?

____

____

____

____

____

____

____

____

If your core values intersect as they did in the scenario just given, the result could be drastic confusion and questioning of your core identity foundation. If this rigid thinking does not allow for the gray areas of situations to influence your decisions in some way, you could create your own self-doubt and the very things that made sense in your world will be the source of frustrations and uncertainty. The ability to move effectively through the gray areas does not mean that the values that make up your core identity are any less meaningful, it simply means that you are willing to take the human factor into account when considering decisions based on those values.

Use the following activity to practice analyzing the intersection of your core values. Choose two of the five core values you have identified as a part of your core identity. In Figure 5.7, place them on the gray scales next to each other with the value identified in white and the polar opposite identified in black. Show the intersection with a connecting line to demonstrate how the gray area gives meaning to your value. See Figure 5.6 for an example.

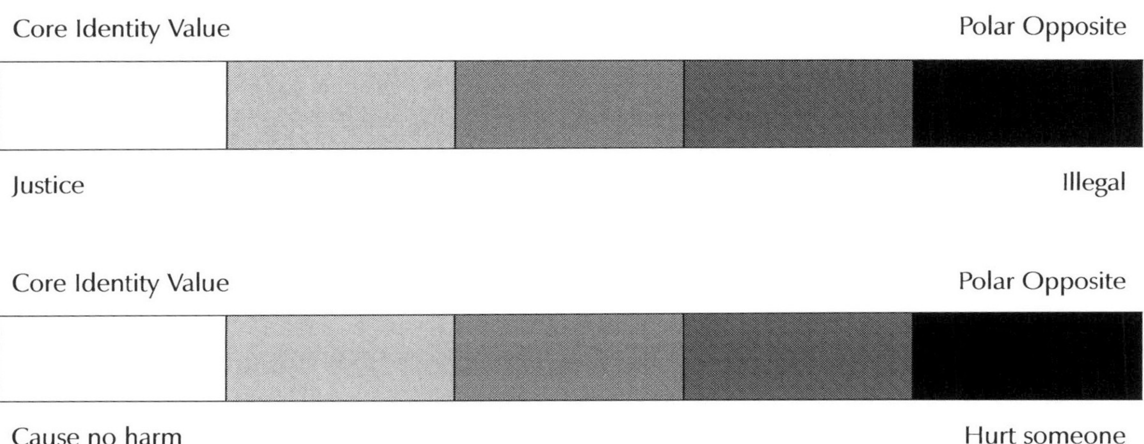

FIGURE 5.6: THE INTERSECTION OF YOUR CORE VALUES (EXAMPLE)

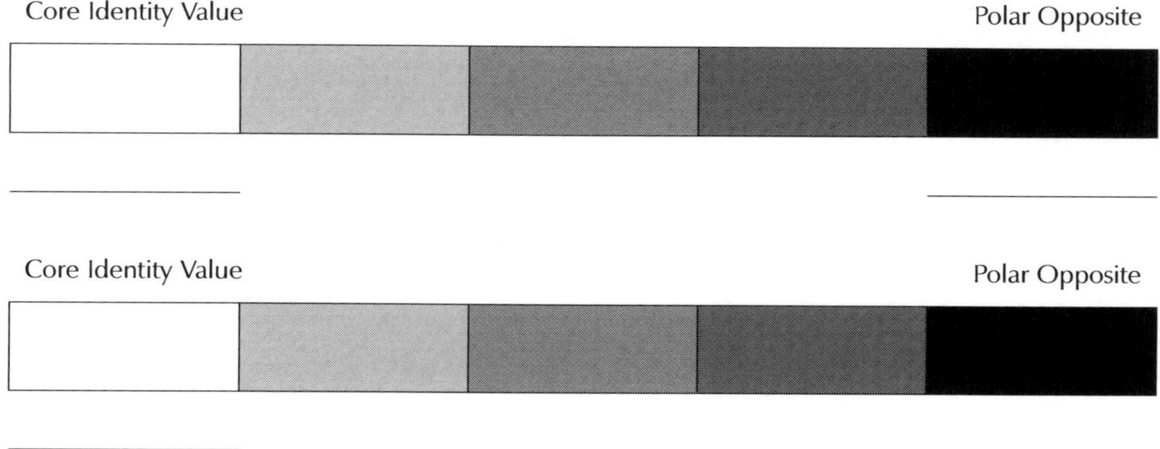

FIGURE 5.7: THE INTERSECTION OF YOUR CORE VALUES

Throughout this chapter you have had the opportunity to explore the values that make up the foundation of who you are as a person. This foundation of core values is referred to as your core identity. One of the strength areas associated with having ASD is the ability a person has to stay true to his or her core identity without giving in to peer pressure, financial pressure, or political pressure, but it is vital to be responsible in identifying and managing this core value commitment.

As with anything, if you allow excesses, you can have a negative impact. This is also true of adhering to your core identity features. These values have a great impact on your life, how you approach relationships, and how you make important decisions. If you allow yourself to carry these values to excess, they will have an impact in those areas as well, but they will most often be negative. Carrying your value to the excess could cause you to damage relationships with others and could contribute to anxiety in your life.

Finally, as a person with ASD, if you subscribe to black-and-white thinking in regard to the values that make up your core identity, you are not respecting the necessary flexibility within the gray area. This gray area represents all the subtle nuances that go along with the human condition. A secondary result of this black-and-white style of thinking is the possibility of the awkward and confusing intersections that may occur between core identity features. In the event that two values come into conflict with each other, you will be forced into the uncomfortable situation of deciding which core identity feature has the most value to you.

BACK TO BASICS

Consider these guiding questions as you prepare to evaluate yourself.

B	**Behavior**	Are you recognizing when you are calm, passionate, and anxious? Do you outwardly demonstrate your core value features? Are you aware of how situations are not always black and white? Are you monitoring the ways your core values intersect? Are you committed to the values you have identified?
A	**Academics**	Are you attending all your classes on time? Are you applying organizational strategies? Are you consistently using your organizational system? Are you keeping up with everything?
S	**Self-care**	Are you getting enough sleep? Are you eating healthily? Are you planning for your self-care activities? Are you keeping your space clean? What are you doing to make sure you are managing your stress level?
I	**Interaction**	Are you checking in with your support team? Are you planning time for social activities? Are you actively engaged in classes? What are you doing to get to know your roommates? Are you checking your email/blackboard daily?
C	**Community**	Do you feel like you belong? Are you asking for help when needed? Have you met anyone new? Do you know the names of any classmates? Are you involved in anything socially?
S	**Self-monitoring**	Are you managing your time? Are you accepting critical feedback? Are you managing your frustration level? Are you willing to see the perspectives of others? Are you advocating for yourself?

BACK TO BASICS: RATE YOURSELF

B	**Behavior** 1 2 3	**Comments**
A	**Academics** 1 2 3	**Comments**
S	**Self-care** 1 2 3	**Comments**
I	**Interaction** 1 2 3	**Comments**
C	**Community** 1 2 3	**Comments**
S	**Self-monitoring** 1 2 3	**Comments**

GOALS

Personal:

Academic:

Social:

Chapter 6

SOCIAL RULES AND SOCIAL CONFUSION

The confusion lies in what is hidden.

INTRODUCTION

Interacting with many diverse people as a college student is unavoidable. For many students, there is a significant transition not only in academic work when they enter college but also when it comes to establishing and maintaining relationships, reacting to social confusion, and advocating for their own needs. Neurotypical students experience this too to some degree. While some social skills might seem to come naturally for neurotypical students, learning to adapt those skills to new contexts is something almost everyone experiences. There is a certain degree of adjusting to and recognizing social norms in college for almost every student.

Students who have ASD will be expected to interact socially in many different ways throughout college. For students with ASD, the process of recognizing their strengths and core values, discussed in previous chapters, is an important process as it provides students with insight that will help them develop a sense of social purpose at college. From engaging in small talk with a new roommate to presenting major research findings in front of professors and classmates, social interaction at the college level occurs with a great variety. Students can depend on some basic social strategies to navigate confusion, especially when they are focused elsewhere, like on maintaining a high standard in their academic work.

Understanding the purpose of social interaction for young adults in the college setting is the first step for students looking for a few "go-to" strategies that can alleviate much social confusion. Social interaction can be unexpected in manner and timing on a college campus, so having a solid understanding of how to assess situations and apply a certain strategy can be an asset. It would be very difficult to create or memorize an exhaustive list of potential college-related social situations and a specific and appropriate response to each situation. With this in mind, students can learn five rules that can be applied to social situations to help understand social confusion and also to help avoid it.

The five Rules of Social Engagement we will discuss in this chapter include:

1. First impressions are vital.
2. Manners matter.
3. People act differently depending on whom they are with.
4. Every person with whom you interact has something significant to offer.
5. Relationships are dynamic.

Students will begin shifting focus in the next chapter to team-building in an intentional career-driven approach to college that is highly dependent on working with others to understand and work through the career preparation process. Having a solid grasp of some fundamental rules will not only help students with peer relationships and academic-based interactions early on in the college experience, but also with career preparation as students begin actively pursuing internships and networking relationships. With an array of new settings and contexts to explore in college, there are some basic skills that will help students address new situations. Through the process of recognizing context and appropriate social behavior and the development of a social first aid kit, intended to serve as a quick-solving social solution field guide, and a response diagram to guide reactions when social miscues occur, career-bound college students with ASD can use simple approaches to common social occurrences at college.

LESSON 1: SOCIAL CONFUSION AND ESTABLISHING PURPOSE

Before we begin exploring the role of social confusion in students with ASD in college and establishing a purpose for learning new social skills, let us first make a point about identity. Students with ASD can struggle with the process of gathering information about new social contexts and social strategies. Social awareness does not demand that you lose sight of who you are—your core values, idiosyncrasies, strengths, and identity—but instead that you simply recognize how effectively interacting socially on campus matters and that social connectedness is, in fact, a beneficial tool despite the inherent unpredictability (Grandin and Barron 2005). The goal should be knowing what your strengths and values are and realizing that while these do not need to change, social awareness and connections to other people are necessary for you as a young adult at college. Having a sense of the pieces of social interaction that are difficult for you guides you purposefully to some strategies to help navigate that element of social interaction.

Preparing for a career while you are a student is an endeavor involving a significant amount of social interaction, not only that which is geared toward pursuing a career, but also peer interaction and intentional interaction with instructors and university staff. It is not surprising that this increase in social demands and the evolving transition in social intentions can produce significant social confusion for students on the spectrum. Gaining a better understanding of the social world around you will serve to help you project your personality and identity through appropriate behavior and discussion. Students who can adeptly negotiate the social atmosphere will be able to ensure that their valuable and unique input is heard and acknowledged, which is crucial for students who are beginning to prepare for a career after college.

Since social rules are cultural constructs, they are not universal truths. Social rules are your culture's unspoken guidelines for interacting with one another. These guidelines might shift from region to region or culture to culture. A polite gesture in one area might be an insult in another. There are social rules for the same behavior, like laughing, in different settings, like a funeral or a party. As a student with ASD, you might find the lack of patterns in social rules frustrating. When expectations for social interactions are unmet, social confusion can happen.

To mediate social confusion, there are a few overall guidelines you can use. There are many sensitive topics about which you can make a note to "proceed with caution." These can include political views, religious beliefs, body-related topics, attitudes about controversial social topics such as sexual orientation or abortion, and public personal rants. As a general rule, students will need to be careful about engaging socially regarding a special interest or area of significant passionate views with anyone who has an opposite view. For example, if a student feels very strongly about a certain political candidate, it would be wise to be cautious when discussing politics with someone who campaigns for the opposing candidate. When it comes to social confusion, though, you also need to note your audience when considering a discussion of taboo topics. It can be confusing to understand why, for example, you can discuss your religious views with your family but need to be careful when discussing your views around your roommate who does not share the same beliefs. The next lesson has a discussion of how dynamic relationships can be.

To illustrate how social confusion happens, the cartoon images below will tell the story of Ben, a college student with ASD, as he acknowledges and reacts to a miscue.

Take a look at the cartoon strip below and think about what behaviors Ben exhibits. Then reflect on the process he goes through to create a solution to his social miscue. Ben's social miscue, initial reaction, solution, and recharge method will be discussed following the image.

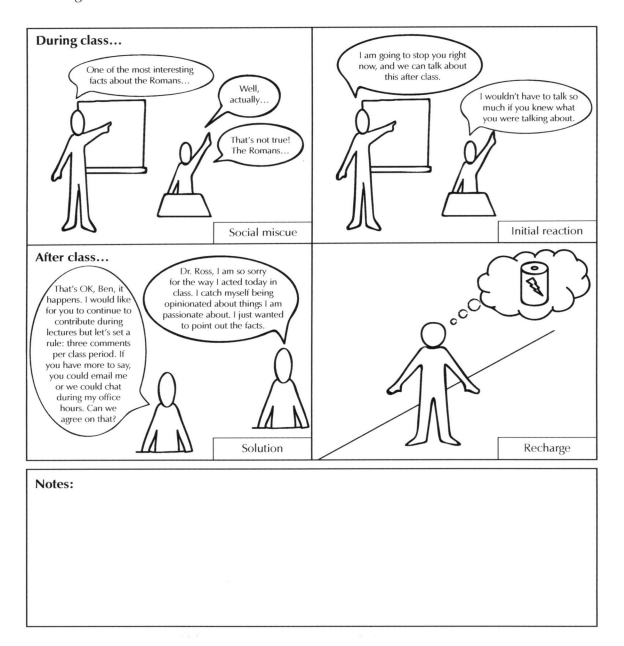

Notes:

SOCIAL MISCUE

In the first box of the strip, Ben, a second-year college student, attends his World Civilizations course. Since Ben has a special interest in ancient Roman civilizations, he has quite a lot to say in class when his instructor, Dr. Ross, lectures on the impact of Roman innovation. After Ben impulsively shouts out interjections and comments throughout the class without being called upon, Dr. Ross loses his temper and yells at Ben in front of the whole class.

Ben's passion for history should be a great benefit to him while attending a World Civilizations course. While his comments were accurate and interesting, a social miscue occurred when he failed to recognize that his behavior in class was distracting. Social miscues like Ben's can occur when context and appropriate behavior is not identified. Some miscues are relatively minor, like interrupting your roommate while he or she is talking, while others are more serious, like misunderstanding the scope of a joke until it is interpreted as a threat to someone's safety.

INITIAL REACTION

When Dr. Ross reprimands Ben in class, everyone else in the room looks at him and he realizes that he had been the only one speaking up in class. Ben is embarrassed, so he snaps back with a snarky comment: "I wouldn't have to talk so much if you knew what you were talking about!"

Ben's initial reaction only made the situation in the classroom worse. The behavior you exhibit immediately after a social miscue is interpreted by those around you. You will need to remember that your reaction after a miscue can impact how difficult it is for you to reach a solution to the social miscue. First impressions from those around you might be assessed quickly following your initial reaction to a miscue. You will learn more about specific social rules like monitoring first impressions in Lesson 2.

SOLUTION

After Ben's initial reaction, the rude comment to Dr. Ross, the instructor ignores Ben and resumes his lecture. Meanwhile, Ben decides to approach Dr. Ross after class to apologize for the disruption. When the lecture finishes, Ben works individually with Dr. Ross to set up a guideline for appropriately contributing to class discussions. They decide that Ben must be called on before speaking and that after three comments in each class, he will have to save all other comments or questions until the next class or send them in an email directly to the instructor.

When social confusion happens, figuring out a solution is a process. You have to consider how or if you will explain your social miscue and then develop a procedure that results in a solution to any consequences from your social miscue or your initial reaction to it. In many instances, positive communication is an effective solution-seeking method. Before your behavior or reaction is explained, your audience makes their own interpretation, leaving room for misunderstandings and more social confusion. While the solution will vary with each instance of social confusion, it is important to remember how the solution was developed. Your social first aid kit later in this chapter will help you organize these solution strategies.

RECHARGE

To recharge after the taxing instance of social confusion during his World Civilizations class, Ben goes on a walk. He has found that walking a familiar path through campus allows him some time to reflect. Thinking about what happened in class, Ben realizes during his walk that he had prevented the rest of his classmates from hearing the lecture material that will appear on the next exam. Now that he has made the connection between his instructor's response and his social miscue, he makes a mental note of the purpose of the new classroom contribution guidelines.

Taking some time to recharge after a situation that causes social confusion can be a beneficial practice for you. Recent sensory overload and general anxieties can be alleviated when you intentionally take time to pause and reflect. For some, like Ben, a recharge technique will be taking a walk. Others might play video games, listen to music, or simply sit alone in their bedroom. It does not matter so much how you recharge as this will be different for every person, but choosing to recharge regularly, and especially after an instance of social confusion, allows you to find closure to situations and prepare to move past tough situations.

CREATE YOUR OWN SOCIAL COMIC

Reflect on a time when you made a social miscue. Create your own story in the comic strip boxes for each step of this process. You can draw a comic or write about your experience.

Social miscue	Initial reaction
Solution	Recharge

Notes:

LESSON 2: RULES OF SOCIAL ENGAGEMENT

It is very possible that people with ASD would rather complete work tasks, study or do recreational activities in isolation. This preference is not necessarily due to the person choosing not to engage with others socially, but can be attributed to the social confusion that often interferes with successful interactions. Whether people with ASD have had negative experiences, become easily frustrated with group members, or have offended people in the past, the end result is shared, an existing confusion about social engagement.

Many of the social cues that neurotpycial individuals follow easily are hidden and not so obvious to people with ASD. These unwritten rules can be the keys to social success or struggles in the social world. Although it is not easy to navigate these rules when you struggle with deciphering them in the first place, it is not impossible to be socially successful. As a person with ASD, you do not have to try to be a social detective in every situation; nevertheless, you must have an awareness of what is happening around you. If you had to analyze every social situation and define the rules to follow in each interaction, the process of engaging with another person could prove to be confusing and exhausting. To help navigate this process, there are a few primary rules that you can follow in any situation that will not lead you astray.

The following Rules of Social Engagement are positive and helpful in any situation. If you keep these rules in mind during any social interaction, you will have a broader opportunity for social success. While none of these rules are absolutes, you will have a greater advantage in social, academic, or work settings if you use these as a guide than if you do not employ any strategy to frame your interactions.

1. FIRST IMPRESSIONS ARE VITAL

When you meet someone for the first time, you never know how important that person could be in your life. You never know if the person you are meeting for the first time could end up being a teaching assistant for your lab course, a potential internship supervisor, a partner on a class project, or even a professor that you do not know yet. The impression you leave in your initial interaction could frame your future interactions with that person.

Take, for example, this scenario: you are in the building for your Chemistry class getting prepared to enter for the first day of lab. As you start to walk into the room, you lift your head and run into a woman entering the room at the same time. You respond in a very condescending and rude way, telling the woman that she should watch where she is walking or she is going to hurt someone or damage lab equipment. She then proceeds into the room and walks to the front of the lab and introduces herself as your lab instructor. This brief interaction could easily define how your semester will turn out. Because you left a negative first impression, this lab instructor could choose not to interact with you in a helpful way, could refuse to spend extra time with you to explain points of confusion, and could have an impact on your course grade.

The idea that your first interaction could determine the direction of your relationship is not to say that things cannot be repaired. If you do leave a negative first impression on someone, typically, people will give someone a second chance to make another impression, but it is not easy to change the first impression. To change a negative first impression, you would have to do twice as much work and be even more respectful and nice to be able to change the impression someone has of you. It isn't as if you can just start over with a person. If you have already left a negative impression, it is like you have already dug yourself a hole and you will need to do a lot of work to be on level ground again.

Write about a time when you left a negative first impression. Did this impact you in any way?

____

____

____

____

____

____

____

2. MANNERS MATTER

We have all heard about how important it is to treat others how we would like to be treated. Some people even refer to this as the golden rule that if followed will give others the impression that we live our lives ethically. This idea of reciprocity in relationships can, however cause significant confusion for people with ASD. Instead of treating others as you would like to be treated, perhaps a better rule to follow is to always use good manners.

Good social manners include things as simple as saying please and thank you, or not passing gas in front of other people. These social manners could also include apologizing if you offend someone, not interrupting others, and not touching anyone or their belongings without permission. By placing importance on the impact you have on others in social situations, you can begin to define your manners that matter to you.

Develop a list of the top three examples of good manners you can commit to in each interaction you have with other people.

1. ______________________________

2. ______________________________

3. ______________________________

3. PEOPLE ACT DIFFERENTLY DEPENDING ON WHOM THEY ARE WITH

People with ASD tend to always stay true to who they are. There is no guessing when it comes to how people with ASD approach and interact with others. In the previous chapter about strengths, the characteristics of honesty and infallible inner character free from peer pressure were identified as primary strength areas that many people with ASD possess. While this is a strength, this is not always how to best navigate social situations.

The way people approach, communicate with, and respond to a person depends largely on the role the other person plays in their life. For example, you can tell a joke that may be a little "off color" to someone you consider a friend, but you would not want to tell that same joke to someone who is your direct supervisor. While you want to stay true to who you are, you will need to adjust your interactions with others depending on who the person is and what role they play in your life.

The idea of people shifting the way they behave based on whom they are interacting with is a confusing one for people with ASD. This social rule does not represent people being fake or manipulative, it is simply a way to engage appropriately with people out of respect. Neurotypical people may shift easily from one social interaction to the other with little cognitive effort, but this may not be the case for a person with ASD. This act of social shifting may take some planning and processing prior to engaging in social situations, but along with anything that is worth mastering, it is worth the practice so this rule becomes one you can follow consistently.

To practice this rule, complete the following charts to show the different ways you would address people. (The first chart is already completed to give you some examples.)

GREETINGS

EXAMPLE:

Friend	Classmate	Professor	Supervisor
Hey, what's up?	Hi John, how did you do on that last test?	Good morning, Dr. Smith.	Good morning, I clocked in and plan to...

Develop your own greeting statement for someone representing these social roles.

Friend	Classmate	Professor	Supervisor

Practice how these social interactions could be different depending on the person with whom you are engaging socially.

ASKING A QUESTION

Friend	Classmate	Professor	Supervisor

GETTING CLARIFICATION ON A DIRECTIVE

Friend	Classmate	Professor	Supervisor

TELLING A JOKE

Friend	Classmate	Professor	Supervisor

4. EVERY PERSON WITH WHOM YOU INTERACT HAS SOMETHING SIGNIFICANT TO OFFER

It is far too often the case that a person with ASD struggles with a group project because he or she does not value the input of the other group members. Whether this is because he or she has a vast amount of knowledge about the topic or because he or she views the other group members as work-shy, this approach to others can significantly interfere with the social experience. This rule of engagement can even be attributed to interactions that could be viewed as insignificant with people that may appear to have no meaningful bearing on his or her life immediately.

Whether you are working on a group project for a class or on a work team for your career, every member of that group is working toward the same goal. Each person has a set of strengths that can contribute to the successful completion of the project. While the person with ASD may contribute significant topic-based knowledge, other members also have knowledge to contribute. In addition, other people may have strength in areas where others do not and this variation is what makes the group successful.

Another thing to keep in mind is that any interaction you have with someone could have bearing on a future request. The person with ASD must monitor all interactions regardless of how seemingly meaningless they may be. It is highly likely that a person with whom you may interact will have something you need assistance with in the future. Take for example, a professor for a college course who may not be a good professor according to how a person with ASD defines a good professor. That person may ask the professor questions that attempt to point out inadequacies and may respond in a condescending tone. These interactions have already set up how the professor views the student with ASD and when that student genuinely needs clarification on something at a later date, the professor may be less likely to offer extra support for the student with ASD.

How has this rule of engagement affected you in the past?

____

____

____

____

____

____

____

____

____

____

5. RELATIONSHIPS ARE DYNAMIC

Perhaps one of the most difficult rules of engagement deals directly with the changes that naturally occur in relationships. As relationships are defined and redefined, the social expectations also shift. A person that could be defined as a boyfriend/girlfriend could easily shift back to the status of friend. If that shift happens, the social interactions with that person must also shift. The same could be said for a friend who gets promoted at work and becomes your supervisor. While at work, the social interaction must be different from when you are engaged in a more social setting.

A person with ASD may have a difficult time understanding how to make the shift in social requirements based on the various types of relationships when the person has not changed. This rule of engagement is based more on the definition of the relationship than on the person involved. Although the person is the same, the expectations change with the role shift. By defining potential social roles and the social expectations associated with each of those roles, you can develop a stronger grasp of the expectations and practice using them in various situations.

In the following activity, potential social roles are defined for you. For each of these social roles, work with a social mentor (a trusted person who understands ASD and can serve as an interpreter of social rules) to develop the expectations associated with the role. (The first is already completed to give you an example.) By developing these expectations for yourself in social situations, you can decrease the possibilities of social miscues.

ROLE DEFINITIONS AND SOCIAL EXPECTATIONS

ACQUAINTANCE

ROLE DEFINITION

This is a person whom you may have met on occasion. You may share a class with this person and possibly know his or her name, but you know very little other personal information. You do not know this person's belief system, political views, family or friends. This person would not be defined as a friend.

SOCIAL EXPECTATION

Because you know very little about this person, it is the safest option to engage in polite conversation free from topics about politics, religion, or sexual orientation. Jokes should all be respectful and you should follow all the Rules of Social Engagement strictly.

FRIEND

ROLE DEFINITION

This person is someone you know well and they know you equally well. You know about their views and preferences regarding many things and you have both shared personal information about yourselves with each other.

SOCIAL EXPECTATION

BOYFRIEND/GIRLFRIEND

ROLE DEFINITION

This person is someone you know intimately. You know details about his or her personal life, you know about his or her family and you enjoy spending time together. He or she trusts you and you have equal trust in this person.

SOCIAL EXPECTATION

HIGHER EDUCATION PROFESSIONAL

ROLE DEFINITION

This person can be your professor, a mentor, a support person, a tutor, an advisor, or any other professional that works in college. This is a professional relationship and can be challenging at times. Although you may enjoy spending time with this person, this is not a personal relationship.

SOCIAL EXPECTATION

SUPERVISOR

ROLE DEFINITION

This person is your boss at your job. He or she has an impact on your employment status. If you have a negative interaction with this person, you could lose your job. This is the most important professional relationship you will have.

SOCIAL EXPECTATION

Understanding the hidden social rules that neurotypical people naturally understand takes significant work for people with ASD. This could cause people with ASD to choose to disengage socially instead of doing the hard work to try to decipher the social puzzle. As a person with ASD, you can adopt these five Rules of Social Engagement as your baseline for social rules. If you follow these rules in all situations, practice the application of these rules, and revisit them frequently, you will reduce the possibility of being offensive socially. This can have a positive impact on your ability to work with others both in school and at work. These rules of engagement can also improve your relationships with friends, family and potential partners by increasing the attention you give to the respect you show others.

LESSON 3: BUILDING YOUR SOCIAL FIRST AID KIT

As people move through life experiences, unfortunate events take place occasionally. While driving down the road, it is possible that a driver will run over a nail and get a flat tire. In this situation, it would be helpful for that driver to have a tool kit in the car to be able to jack up the car, remove the flat tire, and replace the tire with a spare. Without those tools, that situation could not be resolved without calling a professional mechanic. In another setting, a hiker could be taking a new trail and trip over a rock, cutting his hands and legs. In this situation, it would be helpful for the hiker to have a first aid kit in his backpack so he can clean the wounds, apply an antibiotic cream, and cover the wound so it does not get infected. Again, without this first aid kit, the situation could not be resolved without going to a professional medical provider.

In both of these situations, the preference is for people to have the necessary tools available to be able to resolve the situations on their own. The ability to solve difficult situations without depending on others is the key to living independently. Life is full of obstacles and mistakes, but knowing how to solve these difficulties can reduce the possibility of these negative circumstances having a lasting effect.

In social situations, it is also helpful to have a kit of things available to help in difficult situations. This social first aid kit can come in handy when entering a social situation or at the first sign of a social miscue. By depending on the tools that are developed and practiced, the task of managing social interactions can become less exhausting. Your social first aid kit should include the tools we will introduce you to in the following set of activities as well as any previous tools you have learned in the past. Your first aid kit will be personal to you, but as with any tool, this social first aid kit will only be effective if you practice your tools and use them appropriately when you need them. The following five tools are the introductory tools to start building your first aid kit. Add to this kit as you learn new strategies and practice using them frequently.

SOCIAL CONSULTANT

A consultant is generally described as a person with a wide range of knowledge in a particular area who can offer expert advice and guidance to foster growth and understanding. A social consultant is someone who understands the nuances of social situations but also understands how potential miscues can happen for a person with ASD. This person can be a higher education professional, a mentor, a friend, or a family member. The only qualification for being a social consultant is the ability to listen patiently and give honest feedback that can contribute to the growth of the person with ASD.

As a person with ASD, this social consultant must be someone you can trust because you will be sharing information that could be sensitive to you. You will need to be open with this person as you work through dissecting the social miscues that may occur. This person will need to be an open-minded person who can suspend judgment and listen actively to your description of the events. Your social consultant will need to understand that his or her role is to help guide you in the discovery of a solution, not simply solve the situation for you. It is also imperative that your social consultant can remove his or her emotional reaction to your frustrations as you dissect the scenario. Finally, your social consultant must be able to recognize both the larger themes of social situations as well as the finite nuances of each situation as he or she helps you understand the miscues as well as develop solutions to resolve any residual social damage.

SOCIAL CONSULTANTS

Brainstorm some potential people in the various areas of your life that could fill the role of social consultant. Identify them by name and write down the personal qualities that would make them a good candidate to fulfill this support role for you.

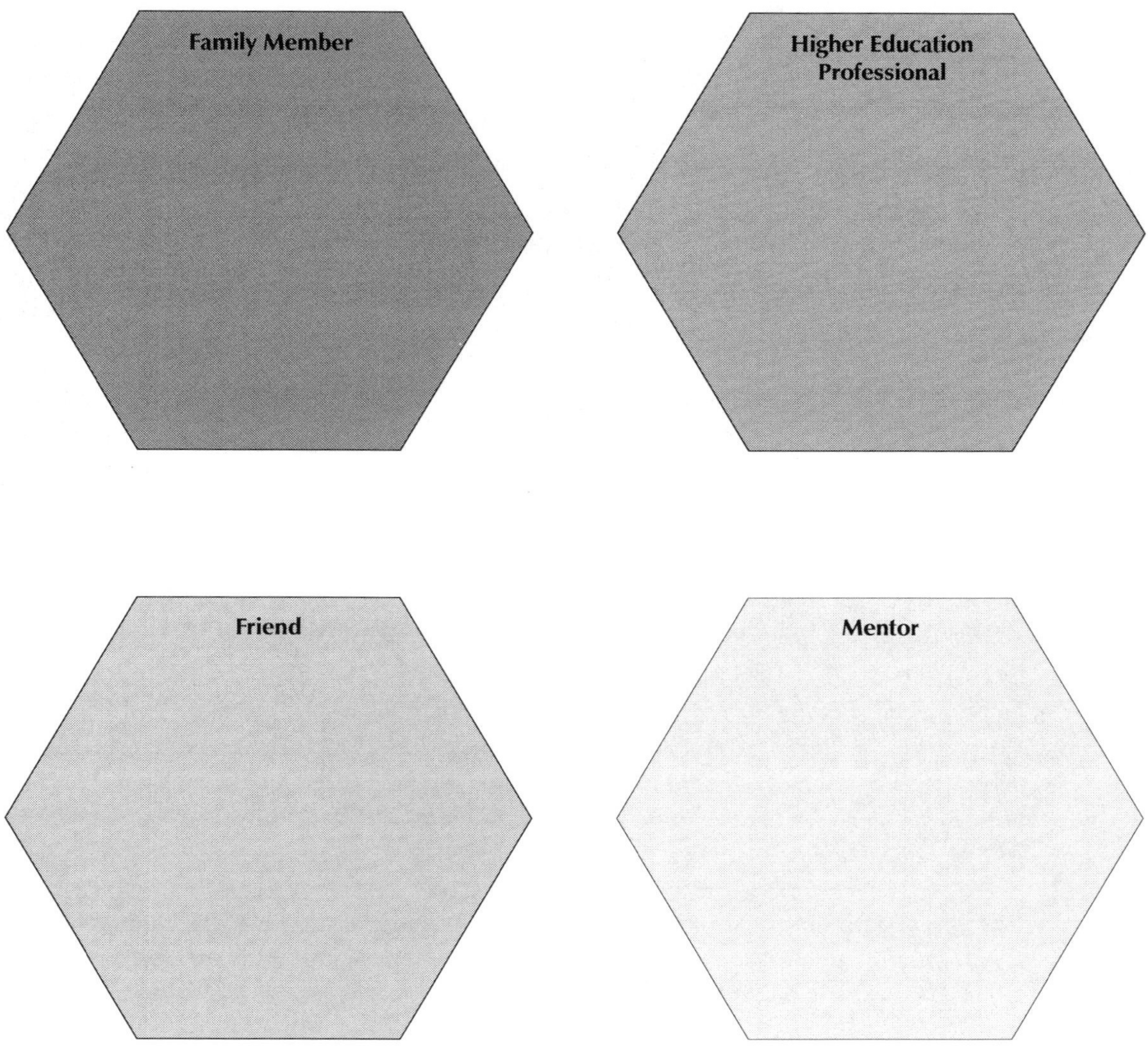

SOCIAL STUDY GUIDE

In many college courses, the content taught is isolated to the lecture, but students must do significant studying independently to gain a strong understanding of the material. This act of independent studying is a difficult habit to develop, but when mastered, can contribute to academic success. Students often develop study guides for courses that look differently for each student. Some students choose to use visual notes to identify key concepts while others use flashcards to study those same concepts.

The same can be said for studying social strategies. As you progress through social situations, it will be important for you to study what is happening around you. Take notes on how people enter conversations, how many times other students ask questions in class, how people show interest in others, how people disagree respectfully with others, etc. These notes will help you develop your social study guide. Depending on your learning style, you can develop these social study guides in several ways. For the purpose of this activity, we will focus on two distinct study guide strategies: social skills mapping, and social scenario flashcards.

SOCIAL SKILLS MAPPING

A social skills map consists of a main skill connected by several supporting facts. This visual representation can serve as a reminder for any social situations you may encounter.

See Figure 6.1 for an example.

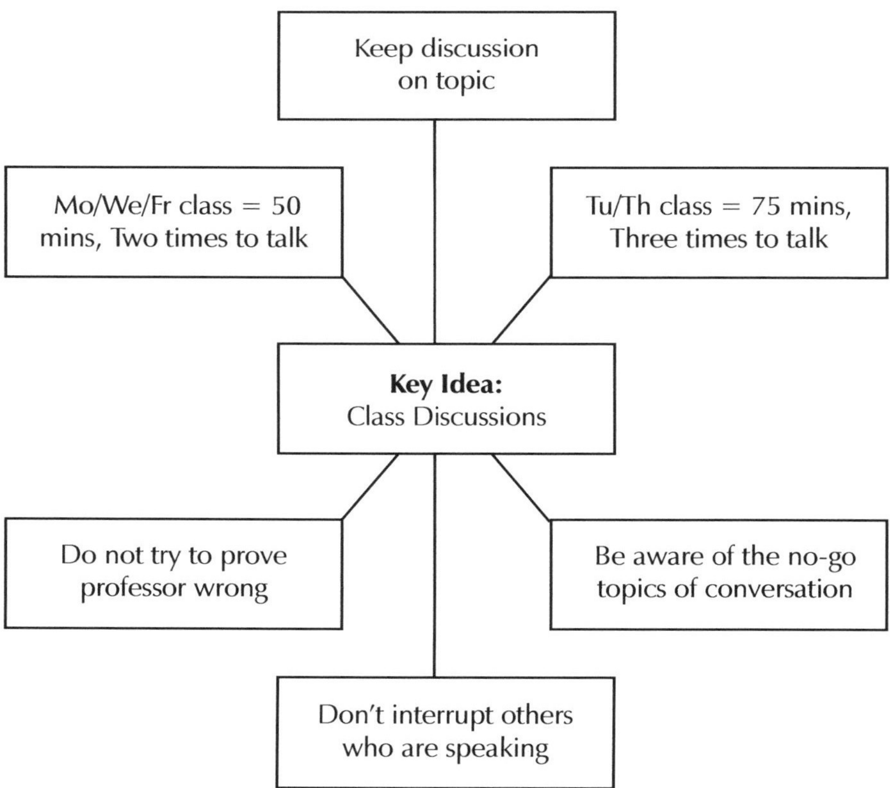

FIGURE 6.1: SOCIAL SKILLS MAP (EXAMPLE)

Now develop your own social skills map with another skill you have observed. Try to outline the most important points of this skill so you can study them and practice consistently.

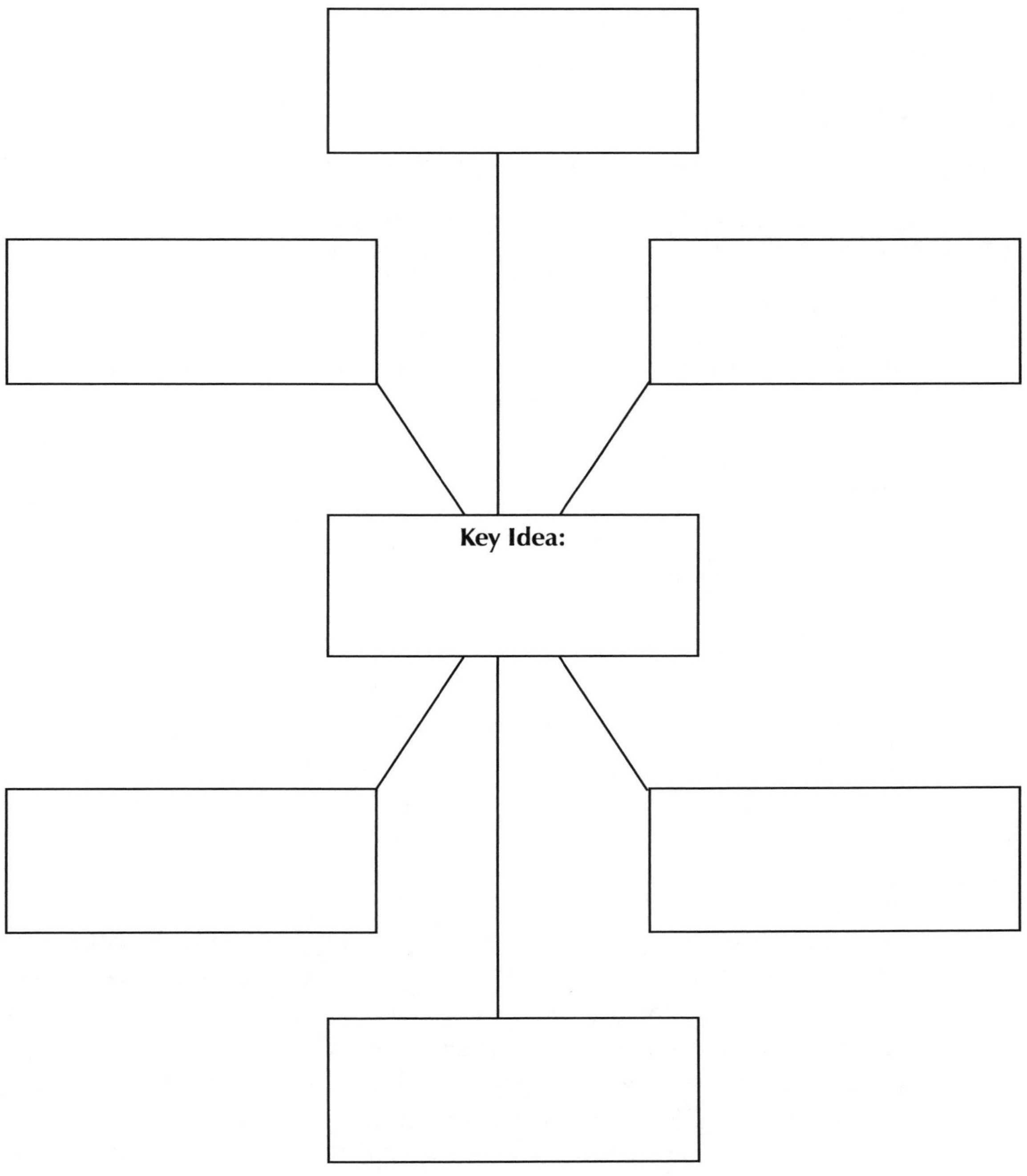

SOCIAL SCENARIO FLASHCARDS

Another way to develop social study guides is to use the same method that students often use to study content in their classes. For social scenario flashcards, write a scenario on the front and a potential tool or solution on the back.

An example is given below.

(FRONT)

As you are leaving your Chemistry class, you overhear a group talking about you. They are talking about how you seem to know all the answers all the time, but can't figure out when to stop talking. They then begin talking about the most recent test and how poorly they think they did on the exam. You are fairly sure you did well, and you could help them, but in light of what they said earlier in the conversation you are just not sure whether you should approach them.

What are some tools you can use? What steps should you take in this scenario?

(BACK)

- Don't engage in the situation right away
- Check in with a social consultant
- Dissect the social situation
- Evaluate the best options for you
- If you choose to offer to help them, write a script for doing so appropriately
- Offer assistance if they choose, and ask them for assistance for social cues

SCRIPTS

Scripts are a method used to help lower the anxiety associate with a variety of social situation (Wolfe, Brown, and Bork 2009). These pre-developed scripts can be used as conversation guides in common situations. These scripts are not intended to guide the entire interaction, but simply give a starting point for a person with ASD to engage. Scripts can initially be developed with the assistance of a social consultant, written on an index card, and read during practice sessions. The hope is that the person will practice the scripts enough so that in a social situation, they can recall the script from memory rather than reading from the physical script.

While scripts can be helpful in many common situations, there are some things to keep in mind when developing and using scripts as a part of your social first aid kit. If you do not practice the scripts and must read from them in social situations, the conversations in which you are engaging will no longer appear authentic. In addition, if you stick to the script too concretely, your interaction will appear "scripted" and robotic, which will also make you appear disengaged in the conversation. Finally, it is impossible to develop a script for every situation you may encounter. It is important to be able to generalize the scripts to various situations. For example, if you develop a script for discussing course content in one class, you should be able to generalize that script for any of your courses.

Work with a partner to pre-develop scripts on index cards and store them in your social first aid kit for practice. If you keep your first aid kit with you at all times, this will allow you to practice your scripts prior to a social interaction allowing you to use them as conversation starters, not guides for the whole interaction.

Please use this example of a script as you begin to pre-develop your own set of scripts with a partner:

> Situation: You are confused about a grade you received on your test and want to ask your professor for clarification.
>
> Script: Approach your professor after class.
>
> Student: "Excuse me, Dr. Smith, I have a question I would like to ask you about the most recent test. Can I talk with you now or would you rather I came to your office hours?"
>
> Dr. Smith: "We can talk now. What do you have a question about?"
>
> Student: "I don't understand why I only received partial credit for question number 14."
>
> Dr. Smith: "I asked in the question for you to show your work, but you have only written your answer. The answer was correct, but you did not show me how you arrived at the answer."
>
> Next steps: At this point, you decide if you want to pursue the conversation further or end the conversation by thanking Dr. Smith for taking the time to clarify and leave the classroom.

To help you practice this skill, pre-develop social scripts regarding the following social situations:

- Ordering food at a restaurant
- Asking a classmate a question about an assignment
- Asking a professor a question about an assignment
- Discussing a difficulty with a roommate
- Asking someone to join you for lunch or dinner

SOCIAL DISSECTION

A scientific analysis of a problem typically involves a dissection of some kind. Whether a scientist is dissecting an animal to study the inner workings of body systems, or dissecting data to try to prove or disprove a hypothesis, the act of dissection is necessary to develop a solution. The same is true for analyzing a social situation and discovering a potential solution to a problem.

When a person with ASD is faced with a new social situation, this experience can be confusing and frustrating. Even with all the tools at hand, it is still possible to become confused by others in the situation and a social mistake can unfortunately take place. In the event that you have offended someone, have become the object of ridicule, or have made someone angry, the best approach to solving the problem is to remove yourself from the situation and the inherent emotions associated with the difficulty. If you attempt to respond in an emotional state, you may not be able to analyze the details effectively through the emotions and may potentially make the situation more difficult to manage.

After you have left the situation, visit with your social consultant to complete your social dissection. This will allow you to objectively analyze the situation and develop a response plan for how you can navigate the response to the people involved. A social dissection can take the form of any other scientific lab manual, which can allow for the step-by-step analysis of the situation. Beginning with a thesis of what happened in mind, use this social dissection form to break the interaction down to the smallest details to discover if your hypothesis about what happened is valid or null.

Reflect on a recent social interaction in which you made a potential social miscue to practice using the process of social dissection. Use the questions on this form as a conversation starter with a social consultant to clarify the potential social miscues and develop a response plan.

Overview of social situation

____

____

____

____

____

____

Hypothesis

____

____

____

What percentage of the time did you spend talking? ________ Listening? __________

Explanation: ____

____

____

What was the topic of the interaction?______________________________

Explanation: ____

____

____

Did you interrupt someone when he or she was speaking? ____________________

Explanation: ____

____

____

Did you discuss no-go topics of conversation? (religion, politics, weapons, sexual identity, etc.) Explanation:____

Did your tone match the tone of the interaction? ____________________________

Explanation: ____

Did you interject an awkward comment? ___________________________________

Explanation: ____

Did you attempt to shift the focus of the interaction?___________________________

Explanation: ____

Did you become argumentative in the social interaction? ________________________

Explanation: ____

Did you attempt to prove someone wrong in the interaction?______________________

Explanation: ____

Did you misread sarcasm or joking in the interaction? __________________________

Explanation: ____

____

____

Was there damage to a relationship as a result of this social miscue? ____________

Explanation: ____

____

____

Did anyone feel threatened or harassed as a result of the interaction? ____________

Explanation: ____

____

____

Examine your initial hypothesis against the answers you provided. Have you proven or nullified your hypothesis? How can you adjust your hypothesis to prove the identified miscue?

____

____

____

____

____

____

____

____

____

____

____

SOCIAL EMERGENCY RESPONSE MANUAL

Emergency management has become a hot topic on college campuses over the last decade. Colleges have developed detailed plans to prepare for and manage any emergency situation on campus as it may arise. These plans typically include a response team, response procedures to specific emergencies, and recovery plans for those emergencies. Although the avoidance of emergencies cannot be guaranteed, the existence of these emergency management plans have made college officials more prepared for the response in case an emergency does happen on their campuses.

A final tool that you can add to your social first aid kit is an emergency response manual. This manual can be a situation-based guide to respond to any social crisis as it may arise. As with a typical emergency response plan, this manual will serve as a quick reference guide to triage a social emergency. The purpose of this guide is the protection of self-confidence, preservation of relationships, and the continuity of daily operations. This guide should include contact information for social consultants, social emergency procedures, and follow-up planning procedures for specific potential social emergencies. To ensure that this manual is an effective tool, study the contents frequently and add to it as needed. This manual should be kept in an easily accessible location at all times.

The format of this manual can take any form you choose, but a consistent approach should be used for any situation. The simple If–Then statements allow for the easy formatting of information and allow the user to flow comfortably from one situation-based response plan to the next in a coherent manner.

SOCIAL EMERGENCY RESPONSE MANUAL

Take some time with a social consultant to develop your personal social emergency response manual. The information in this manual can help you respond appropriately in the moment when a social emergency may arise.

SOCIAL CONSULTANTS

The first step in the resolution of social emergencies is to identify social consultants.

Name:	Contact info:
Name:	Contact info:
Name:	Contact info:

SOCIAL EMERGENCY RESPONSE PLAN (EXAMPLE)

IF	You show up for your Psychology class to find a note on the door from your professor. The note says that the class has moved to the library for the day so students can learn the process of research. You have never been to the library and the note does not say where to meet the class.
THEN	Take a deep breath and calm yourself. Look at your campus map to find the library. If you do not have a campus map, ask someone where the library is. Proceed to the library and ask at the reference desk where your class is meeting. Use specific information in your question. Say, "Where is the Psychology 101 class meeting today?"
RESPONSE	Find your class and join them in the class activities without disturbing the discussion that is occurring.
FOLLOW-UP	Approach the professor after class and let him/her know why you were late for class. Say, "I saw the note on the door and panicked for a minute because I have a difficult time with a sudden change in schedule. I also did not know where the library was or where to meet the class. I solved the problem, but I was late and I am sorry about that. I will try to not let that happen again." Then ask if you missed anything significant in the beginning of the class.

SOCIAL EMERGENCY RESPONSE PLAN

IF	

THEN

RESPONSE

FOLLOW-UP

LESSON 4: DIGGING YOUR WAY OUT

Even with all the tools and supports in place, it is possible still to have a significant social miscue that could have detrimental effects if not managed appropriately. Social interactions may never be easy for a person with ASD. It is more likely that social interactions will always be work, but these interactions and the relationships that accompany them are worth the work.

Reflect on a time when your social miscues have damaged a relationship and made you feel stuck in the situation. When you are stuck in a social hole, you may feel frustrated, overwhelmed, or angry. Regardless of the emotions associated with feeling stuck in this hole, it is vital to identify the details of the situation so you can resolve the social miscue and salvage relationships. Sometimes the process of digging your way out can be a simple process, which includes recognizing the miscue and apologizing quickly. However, depending on the situation, this process can be difficult to navigate, often requiring the support of others.

The first step in digging yourself out of a social hole is to recognize that you have made a social miscue. Once you have recognized that you have fallen in this social hole, analyze the situation in detail. Identify who is involved, how you have impacted those involved, how the situation has impacted you, and any residual effects the situation may cause. Instead of staying stuck in the mud at the bottom of the hole, there are steps you can take to dig your way out. These steps are not linear in nature, but tend to be more cyclical. It is highly likely that you will progress through a step to get out of the hole, but need to revisit a previous step to ensure fluency.

These steps include:

- Acknowledgement
- Communication
- Response
- Re-evaluation
- Moving on.

ACKNOWLEDGMENT

In this initial step, it is important to recognize that a situation exists. Ask yourself what role you play in this situation and how others are impacted. Identify potential consequences for staying stuck in the situation and evaluate the impact of the consequences. Finally, make an informed decision about how to proceed through this step.

POTENTIAL TOOLS FOR PROCEEDING THROUGH THIS STEP

- Identify the misunderstanding by performing a social dissection
- Research the consequences
- Reflect on the consequences
- Discuss with a social consultant

COMMUNICATION

In this step, it is important to frame your communication about the situation that has caused you to be stuck. Because social communication can be difficult for people with ASD, it will be vital for you to proceed through this step with due diligence. Outline your role in the situation and take responsibility for your own behavior. Do not place blame on others at this stage, or you will not be able to progress through the step required to dig your way out.

POTENTIAL TOOLS FOR PROCEEDING THROUGH THIS STEP

- Document your responsibility in the situation
- Engage your social consultant to discuss potential solutions
- Develop a script for communicating with others involved
- Practice your script until you are comfortable discussing the situation

RESPONSE

This third step in digging your way out of the social hole is the one that requires the most work. Once you have identified the details of the situation and communicated about your responsibility in the situation, you must develop a response plan for how you can mitigate the damage that may have occurred. This step includes developing a detailed plan and carrying that plan out effectively.

POTENTIAL TOOLS FOR PROCEEDING THROUGH THIS STEP

- Consult your emergency response manual
- Identify similar situations that are reflected in your manual
- Develop a social emergency response plan
- Identify logical steps to take to complete the plan

RE-EVALUATION

Once you have carried out your response plan, it will be vital to assess the effectiveness of the steps you have taken. Even the most well-thought-out plan can be ineffective if it does not address the actions at the core of the situation. It is important to not only recognize how you feel about the resolution, but also how the other people involved feel about the resolution. The perspective of others is of high priority at this step. At this step, it is common to move backwards in order to develop another plan. Moving backwards in this process is not a negative movement, but a fulfilling movement and a part of the re-evaluating process.

POTENTIAL TOOLS FOR PROCEEDING THROUGH THIS STEP

- Develop a script asking for feedback about the resolution
- Engage your social consultant to reflect on the resolution and/or feedback
- Identify potential holes left unfilled
- Develop a follow-up response plan as needed

MOVING ON

The final step required to dig yourself out of the social hole is to move on. After you have followed all the steps in this model, it is still possible that someone will be upset or not want to engage with you socially. That is the other person's prerogative. You can only be responsible for your own feelings and behaviors. You must forgive yourself and be willing to move forward socially. People do not expect perfection from others so allowing yourself to learn from your social miscues is the best opportunity to move on.

POTENTIAL TOOLS FOR PROCEEDING THROUGH THIS STEP

- Reflect on the resolutions and re-evaluation of the situation
- Identify existing social barriers to getting out of the hole
- Identify whether you own those barriers or if they belong to others
- Develop social study guides to help situations like this in the future
- Forgive yourself and move on

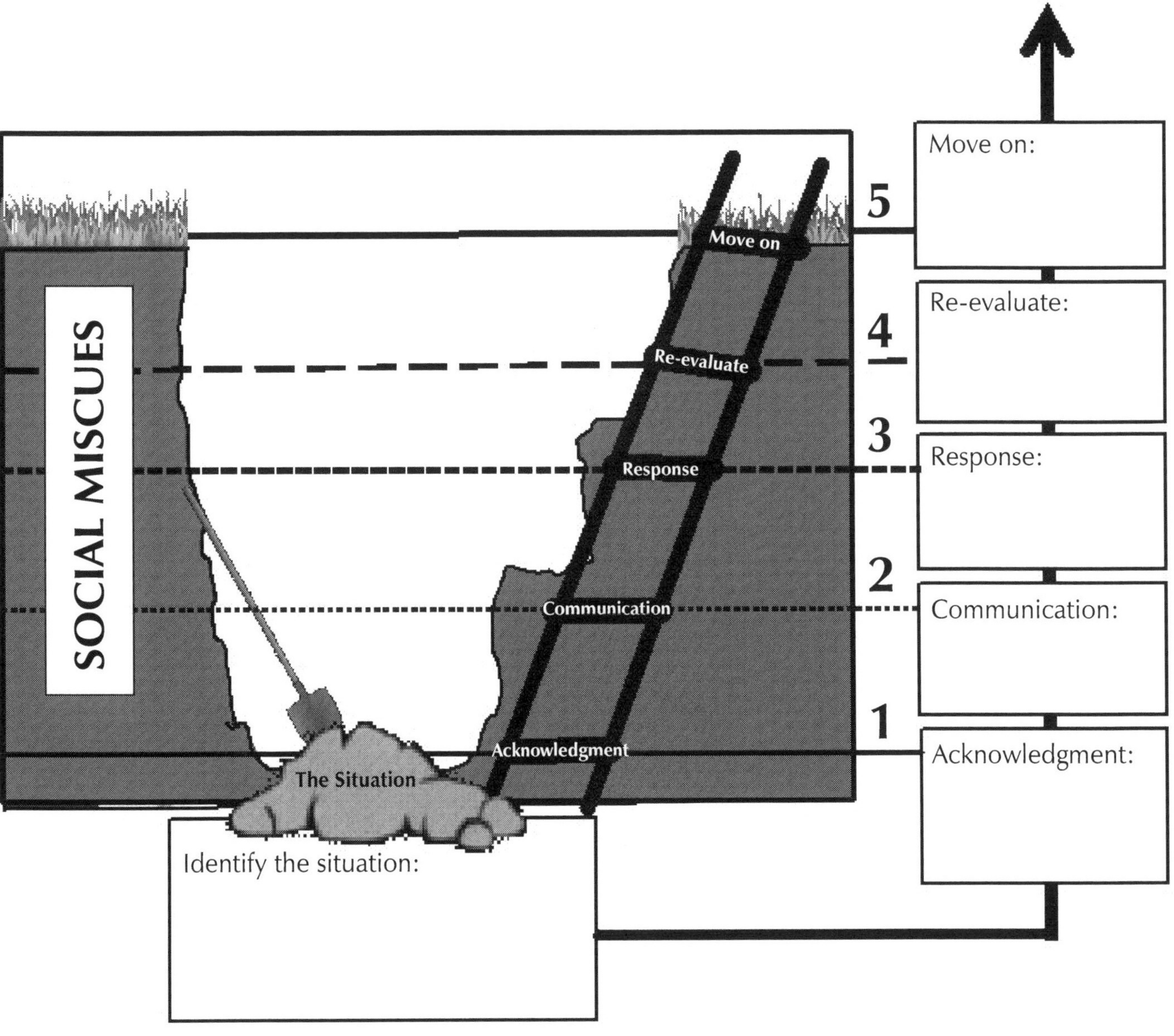

Figure 6.2: Digging Your Way Out

As a college student in a new social environment, at some point you will experience social confusion. Navigating your interactions at college with a solid understanding of social rules allows you to consider what you know about your own potential social miscues and use some strategies to prevent and manage social confusion. As a young adult with ASD, the social transition encountered at college can be as difficult as the academic transition. As you progress through college, you will find that you need to be keenly aware of your social behavior as you prepare for the next step, a career. Being able to transfer your knowledge of social rules and strategies from this chapter to interactions with varying audiences and within varying contexts means that you will be actively practicing for future career-focused social interactions.

Utilizing your understanding of social confusion from Lesson 1, the five Rules of Social Engagement from Lesson 2, the strategies in your social first aid kit from Lesson 3, and the response techniques for digging your way out from Lesson 4 will ensure that you are appropriately equipped for social interactions in college. You will able to acknowledge social confusion and know how miscues occur, you will have problem-solving strategies for gauging social interactions, a guide to "emergency" social miscues, and finally an opportunity to explore what happens when you have fallen into a hole through social mishaps and what you can do to dig yourself out. Keep these techniques and strategies in mind as you interact with your peers, instructors, and anyone else you interact with on campus, and you can navigate social confusion much more efficiently and be prepared for those unexpected social interactions that can lead to confusion. Evaluate your growth in this area on the following BASICS chart.

BACK TO BASICS

Consider these guiding questions as you prepare to evaluate yourself.

B	**Behavior**	Are you communicating effectively with the people around you? Are you aware of social miscues? What do you do to respond to social miscues? Are you using strategies to help with social interactions? Are you learning from having to dig yourself out of social holes?
A	**Academics**	Are you attending all your classes on time? Are you applying organizational strategies? Are you consistently using your organizational system? Are you keeping up with everything?
S	**Self-care**	Are you getting enough sleep? Are you eating healthily? Are you planning for your self-care activities? Are you keeping your space clean? What are you doing to make sure you are managing your stress level?
I	**Interaction**	Are you checking in with your support team? Are you planning time for social activities? Are you actively engaged in classes? What are you doing to get to know your roommates? Are you checking your email/blackboard daily?
C	**Community**	Do you feel like you belong? Are you asking for help when needed? Have you met anyone new? Do you know the names of any classmates? Are you involved in anything socially?
S	**Self-monitoring**	Are you managing your time? Are you accepting critical feedback? Are you managing your frustration level? Are you willing to see the perspectives of others? Are you advocating for yourself?

BACK TO BASICS: RATE YOURSELF

B	**Behavior** 1 2 3	**Comments**
A	**Academics** 1 2 3	**Comments**
S	**Self-care** 1 2 3	**Comments**
I	**Interaction** 1 2 3	**Comments**
C	**Community** 1 2 3	**Comments**
S	**Self-monitoring** 1 2 3	**Comments**

GOALS

Personal:

Academic:

Social:

Chapter 7

BUILDING YOUR TEAM

It takes a team to reach success.

INTRODUCTION

Working with others in some form of co-operative group is a vital part of being a contributing member of a community. Whether that community is a classroom work group or a team of co-workers completing a task together, it will be equally important to be able to manage the process of working collaboratively with others. The concept of working with others to complete a shared goal is a task that is met with disdain and trepidation by many people with ASD. This response to working with a team of people to complete projects could be attributed to many things, but the main reasons discussed by college students with ASD are as follows:

- The need to produce very high-quality work
- Social communication confusion
- Lack of confidence in the ability of the other group members.

People with ASD tend to carry a high level of personal expectation for the work they produce. It is rare to meet a college student with ASD who is content with earning an average grade by doing the least amount of work allowed. Unfortunately, that is not an approach shared by many neurotypical college students. Many students who come to college have the mentality that they want to do what is easy and gain benefit from the least amount of effort. This has been the approach of transitioning college students for years, but this is not a shared approach with the majority of transitioning college students with ASD.

College students with ASD have typically excelled academically throughout their K–12 school years. If they did not do well in specific subjects, it usually was not due to lack of effort. Comments from teachers in high school regarding students with ASD have included thoughts similar to "I wish more students worked as hard as …" or "If … has a task to complete, I know it will be done well and on time." When these sentiments are what students with ASD hear and are defined by throughout middle and high school, they carry these expectations of themselves into college or the work force. The expectation remains that a high level of work will be produced and it will be completed on time to the best of his or her ability. When work groups include others that may not carry the same level of personal expectation, some hesitance about work groups emerges. The truth remains that it is not practical to expect that all group members will carry the same work ethic and commitment for high-quality end products. These variances occur not only because of the dichotomy between ASD and neurodiversity, but for a plethora of other reasons as well. It is not reasonable to expect that all members of any given group will always contribute the highest level of work by the expected due date, but it is also not reasonable to go through college and into a career with the expectation that there will never be a situation requiring task completion through collaborative work.

The social confusion that can easily occur for people with ASD is another reason why working in groups is highly stressful for this population. The notion that not only do individuals have to share in the workload, manage the expectation they place on others, communicate with others about task completion, monitor the process of task completion, and discuss progress as it occurs, but they also must prepare for the social interaction and practice communication to avoid any social miscues that could potentially occur, adds to the overwhelming workload of an individual with ASD. The energy required to manage the social aspect of group work is tremendous and could easily detract from the end product expected from the individual.

The impact of the potential social confusion could be attributed to a person with ASD making social miscues expressing information or the difficulty could lie in the person with ASD receiving social information differently. For example, a person could be assigned to a work group to research and present about the weather pattern shift over the last century. If the group member that has ASD is very interested in this topic, he or she could take over the conversation citing statistics and facts about the shifting weather patterns over the past century without allowing the other members to offer input into what the project should include. This interaction, although unintentional, could turn off the other group members and make them not want to work with individuals with ASD on this project or on any future projects. This act of monopolizing the conversation could translate to the other group members as being egotistical and unwelcoming of the ideas of others.

The impact could also be felt from the opposite direction. In the same project example as above, the group members could gather to begin work and the individual with ASD could begin to share knowledge as stated previously. In this situation, the group members could pick up on the passion and vast knowledge base for the topic and see it as an opportunity to not do any work but claim credit for the project. It is unfortunate that people are willing to manipulate situations like this, but it is possible that a person with ASD could become the workhorse for the group completing all tasks to the highest level of competence and the group could claim credit for the work completed. This could all happen without the individual even reading the social cues that this plan was underway. The confusion with expression or reception of information in group settings can contribute to the aversion to group work, but again, group work is not something that can be avoided. The expectation of a successful individual lies not only with individual success but also with the ability to work with others to accomplish a common goal.

Finally, people with ASD tend to avoid working in groups because they are not confident that other group members will or can contribute the same level of cognitive energy and commitment to the project. This fear might come from past experiences or pre-judging neurotypical peers. This uncertainty about working with others can be categorized into two distinct areas of concern: the concern for the lack of knowledge and the concern for the lack of work ethic.

People with ASD tend to know a lot of information about specific topics, so when it is required to work in a group to fulfill a project goal, this could either be highly beneficial or detrimental to the group process, depending on how the person contributes this knowledge. If the information shared is beneficial to the project and the group members respect the input as presented, this knowledge base could make a significant contribution to the successful completion of the goal. Conversely, if the knowledge is presented in isolation and the other members are not given opportunity to contribute equally, the person with ASD could easily turn the group members off to collaboration and can be viewed as being very condescending. When neurotypical people feel they are being placated, they often will no longer be interested in working with or communicating genuinely with the other person. Although the goal of the group is shared and the knowledge offered by the group member with ASD is vital, if it is communicated inappropriately, the knowledge and contributions of the group member with ASD will not be accepted.

The other area of concern that causes a lack of confidence in other group members points directly to the work ethic of others. If a person with ASD has a task he or she must complete, the task will usually be completed on time and to the best standard possible. Unfortunately, this level of self-expectation is not equally shared among the general population. There are some people who would rather put in the least amount of effort to achieve the goal, and who feel that the timeliness of completion is not of importance. The component of this that causes the distress is the fact that others are given equal benefit for unequal effort. Whether that benefit is a grade, a degree, or a raise at work, if other members of the group do not demonstrate the same commitment and work ethic to the group, the person with ASD views this as dishonest and wrong. The end product of the group is then trivialized and the group member with ASD leaves the group project disillusioned.

While all of these issues are genuine and valid, there is no argument that every person who hopes to experience success will in fact be required to work as a part of a team either in college or in their career. The key to making this a positive and effective experience is for people with ASD to recognize that all members of the team have something to offer to the end result. Whether the contribution is knowledge, organization, or motivation, everyone can contribute something substantial. All members of a team have specific strengths and preferences for interaction. The ability to recognize these preferences and utilize that information to facilitate the completion of the task requires analyzing the actions and reactions of the other group members. Considering the strengths associated with analytical behaviors of people with ASD, this task could potentially lead to the decrease of anxiety related to working as a part of a team to complete a task.

LESSON 1: UNDERSTANDING YOUR PREFERENCES

The first step in being able to analyze the preferences of other group members is to be able to analyze and respect your own preferences. Once a person can identify his or her own preferences in group participation, the building of a team can commence. A successful team is made up of individuals that complement the strengths of each other, not share the same strengths and weaknesses. To position a team for success, it is important to understand the contributions of each member starting with yourself. Use the following tool to analyze your preferences.

SELF-PREFERENCE ANALYSIS

To assist in identifying your individual preferences and the strength of preference associated with each area, read each statement pair and choose the one with which you most identify. Once you have identified a preference between each pair, tally the number of responses for each side and circle the tallies on the number line under each side. Each preference area can be a spectrum that can shift depending on the task and the person with whom you are working. As a baseline, consider a class activity that requires you to communicate and plan with at least one other person as you complete this analysis.

EXTROVERTED VS. INTROVERTED

E	I
☐ I like being around a lot of people	☐ It takes a lot of energy for me to be in large groups
☐ I like having many acquaintances	☐ I would rather have a few very close friends
☐ I can start a conversation with anyone	☐ It is hard for me to join a conversation
☐ I get energy from being around people	☐ I get energy from being alone and quiet
☐ I would rather be with a group of people than alone	☐ I would rather be alone or with a small group
☐ I enjoy parties and social events	☐ I enjoy movies or small group dinner parties
☐ I am focused on what happens around me	☐ I am focused on what happens within me
☐ I tend to get bored easily when I am alone	☐ I tend to reflect and recharge when I am alone
☐ I tend to get revitalized and recharged when I am with others	☐ I tend to get overwhelmed and tired when I am with groups
☐ I have been described as enthusiastic or talkative	☐ I have been described as reflective or quiet

← →

10 9 8 7 6 5 4 3 2 1 0 1 2 3 4 5 6 7 8 9 10

PRESENT VS. FUTURE

P	F
☐ I think about the current needs	☐ I often think about the end result
☐ I am concerned about meeting short-term goals	☐ I am concerned with meeting the large goal
☐ I want to be able to complete a task today	☐ I can work on tasks over long periods of time
☐ I use daily task lists	☐ I use monthly/semester planning calendars
☐ I feel accomplishment when I complete my daily goals	☐ I feel accomplishment when I can plan strategically
☐ I wait until just before deadlines to start work	☐ I work on long-term projects in defined timelines
☐ I tend to overlook long-term projects	☐ I focus heavily on meeting long-term project goals
☐ I can be described as a task completer	☐ I can be described as an organizer
☐ I enjoy completing projects	☐ I enjoy planning projects
☐ I have been described as an activator	☐ I have been described as a planner

←——————————————————————————→

10 9 8 7 6 5 4 3 2 1 0 1 2 3 4 5 6 7 8 9 10

ANALYTICAL VS. CONTEXTUAL

A	C
☐ I feel comfortable finding results	☐ I feel comfortable making connections
☐ I like working with data	☐ I like organizing findings
☐ I am good working in groups with structure and routine	☐ I am good working in groups that are free thinking and open
☐ I make decisions based on results	☐ I make decisions based on relating information
☐ My strength is in observing details	☐ My strength is in communicating results
☐ I would rather compile statistics	☐ I would rather present results
☐ I learn by analyzing information	☐ I learn by discussing results
☐ I tend to isolate details in problems	☐ I tend to look for linkages in solutions
☐ I can be described as a systemizer	☐ I can be described as a relator
☐ I like working with mathematical equations	☐ I like writing and presenting about results

10 9 8 7 6 5 4 3 2 1 0 1 2 3 4 5 6 7 8 9 10

STRUCTURED VS. FLEXIBLE

S	F
☐ It is important to be on time	☐ I am usually on time
☐ I like having detailed schedules to follow	☐ I typically work best with an open schedule
☐ I am comfortable with defined roles and duties	☐ I am comfortable with flexible role definitions
☐ I like due dates and timelines	☐ Due dates make things stressful for me
☐ I am comfortable when everyone stays on task	☐ I enjoy co-operative sharing of ideas
☐ I get anxious when schedules are disrupted	☐ I can easily adjust to changes in schedules
☐ If people are late I think it is disrespectful	☐ It doesn't bother me if people are late
☐ I enjoy working in a controlled environment	☐ I like an environment where change is frequent
☐ I can be described as systematized	☐ I can be described as adaptable
☐ I would rather be in control of a project	☐ I would rather work in a collaborative group on a project

10 9 8 7 6 5 4 3 2 1 0 1 2 3 4 5 6 7 8 9 10

Developing an understanding of your own strengths and preferences can help you develop an understanding of your role within groups. In the previous pairs of descriptors, you were asked to identify your preferential statement. The intention of this exercise was not to develop a polar preference for each pair, but instead to demonstrate the spectrum of preference for each pair. While you may have strength in each area, it is likely that you will be able to adjust to situations and the people with whom you are working if you are able to analyze their strength areas as well.

In the first pair of descriptors you were asked to identify your preference in statements regarding your interactions with people. The descriptors are identified as extrovert and introvert. An extroverted person is often seen as being friendly and outgoing while an introverted person is seen as shy and withdrawn. While these descriptions may be partially true, they are not complete. There is more under the surface for both extroverted as well as introverted people. There are positive and negative aspects of each preference as well, which is why there are more people that exist somewhere on the spectrum between the two polar opposites.

An extroverted person requires the company of others to be energized. This group can become easily bored when alone and their energy levels become quickly depleted unless they are involved in conversations with others. Extroverts seek out social outlets and often think when they speak. Extroverts engage in social interactions with ease and are concerned with the world external to them. This approach tends to be the typical way people interact with each other, which is why this method of interaction tends to be the social norm. There are strengths associated with this preference in that extroverts are viewed as more socially adept. The goal of this person may be to connect with everyone involved to make sure everyone is comfortable and heard. However, a polar extrovert will often engage with a number of people, but those people can be identified as acquaintances at best. Extroverted people often spend a short amount of time with a lot of people in social situations. While they are masterful at networking and can connect people with ease, they can also be viewed as shallow and flighty and are not often taken seriously in professional situations.

Conversely, an introverted person requires solitude and time to think to be able to recharge their energy. This group of people can become easily overwhelmed in social situations and withdraw to observe and think about the interactions of others. Introverts often seek out quiet time to read, analyze information or simply be alone with their thoughts. The strengths associated with people who relate most as introverted are being adept at thinking and analyzing the impact of what they are about to say before speaking, so they are often viewed as highly intelligent and thoughtful. The goal of this person may be to analyze all the details of a situation before commenting to be able to make the most impact with their limited comments. Because this is not the social norm for how people interact, this group of people is often seen as shy and, occasionally, socially awkward. Introverts are often viewed as having depth and are granted the title of intelligent before contributing anything to the conversation; however, a polar introvert can easily be seen as too laid back and devoid of an opinion. In addition, it is easy for a polar introvert to have their social contribution leveled by an extroverted person. Finally, because of the preference not to engage automatically in a social situation, people who operate as polar introverts can be seen as snobby, rude, or even angry.

In the second set of preference pairs, you were asked to examine statements regarding your focus on timelines. These statements worked to identify whether you are a present-level thinker or future-level thinker. Do you think about the here and now identifying current goals, or do you see the bigger picture and identify strategic goals for the future? As with all of these preference pairs, there is strength and benefit to both. The difficulty arises when a person uses a polar preference and does not allow fluid movement between the two preferences.

A present-level thinker tends to focus on the tasks of the day or week. This person works well in activating and monitoring short-term task completion and is a strong advocate for "To Do" lists. When goals are outlined and success indicators are identified, this person can be a great motivator to complete the tasks on the list. The strength associated with this preference area can be defined as being responsible and effective in the process of task completion. The goal of this person may be to identify the achievable steps for the group so they can have some measured successes. Conversely, if this is a polar preference, this person can be seen as a rigid taskmaster who cannot see the big picture. For any project or program to be successful, a person must be able to plan for the future success. Whether that future success is the completion of a project or the development of a new initiative, if a person is not invested in the planning process, it may be difficult to commit fully to the completion of individual tasks.

The opposite side of this preference pair is a future-level thinker. This person tends to focus on the future plan for the project or program and does well in creating a future ideal for the finished product. When there are open-ended thoughts and proposed ideas, this person can thrive on the creativity and thinking that goes into planning for the future completion. This person often thrives on strategic planning and working with groups that are tasked with creating project goals that align with the big picture of the organization. The strength associated with this preference can be defined as being a visionary who can see the contributions of all members resulting in a great success in the future. The goal of this person may be to generate a large scheme idea which the group can work towards together. Conversely, if a person displays this as a polar preference, this person can be viewed as an idealist who does not think realistically about the details required to reach completion. Neither of these preferences is the "correct" approach to adopt, but moving between each, as the task requires, is the best approach.

The third preference pair you evaluated deals directly with the work you prefer to complete in groups. The statements in this pair addressed whether you would rather analyze information and explore the details of projects thoroughly or contextualize the information and develop methods to synthesize and present findings. In any project, there is a need for both sides of this preference pair and your strength area can help the group reach the end result with great success. The difficulty lies in the inability to recognize the need and validity of the opposite side of your preference.

A person who would choose to work with numbers, complete statistics, and analyze data is often considered highly intelligent. This person can recognize patterns in numbers, see the connections and correlations between data sets that could easily be overlooked by others. This member of the group could be seen as the logical, systemizing individual who will ensure that the data is accurate to support the group's hypothesis. The strength associated with this preference is that of being a detailed thinker who is both intelligent and logical in approach. This person will often be consistent and approachable because there is little emotion involved in their interactions. Conversely, a person who is analytical as a polar preference can often turn people off in the group because they are data driven and do not recognize the emotional needs of the other group members. It could be easy for this person to disregard the importance of other group members and, if not careful, they could offend the other members with comments or condescending attitudes.

The opposite side of this preference pair is the person who prefers to contextualize and synthesize information. The person who prefers to operate in groups in this manner is often seen as a connector who is a good group member and public speaker. This person is possibly highly likable, charismatic, and focuses on ensuring that all members are heard and contributing to the end product. The strength associated with this preference is that of being a person-centered thinker who is able to analyze the contributions of others, synthesize the information, and contextualize the findings into a cohesive end product. The goal of this person is to make sure every member of the group is happy with the final product. Conversely, a person who has this as a polar preference may seem "wishy-washy" and too flexible. If this person does not communicate about his or her contributions to the group, the rest of the group could perceive the input as non-substantial and could become upset that this person is not contributing to the end product equally.

The final preference pair you examined looked at the method in which the group must operate. Regardless of the task at hand, a group must set their own set of group rules to follow together. If you are a person who must have structured guidelines and rules and you are paired with several people who are more flexible in how the work time is organized, it may be very difficult for you to participate in the group process.

A person who has a preference for structured timelines and work assignments may flourish in a group that shares those same goals. It is often very important that group meeting times are outlined ahead of time and the expectation is that everyone will be on time and share the same level of commitment to the end product. The strength of the person who is highly structured is that of the ability to show strong work ethic and commitment to the group rules. The goal of this person may be to keep everyone accountable to the timelines and tasks at hand while ensuring the completion of the group goal. Conversely, if structure is the polar preference, this person could be viewed as obstinate and only concerned with the outlined group rules. If this person is not willing to recognize the potential flexibility of rules, they could turn the group against them quickly without recognizing the potential pitfall.

The opposite end of this preference pair is a person who prefers flexibility in work groups. This person is likely to be comfortable going with the flow when it comes to group rules, guidelines and timelines. He or she may not be overly concerned with all group members being on time to every meeting, or having duties outlined and adhered to for each member. The strength associated with this preference is the ability to work through many difficult group dynamics with grace. The goal of this person may be to keep the peace among group members while working through the tasks required. Conversely, if being flexible with group requirements is a polar preference, this could cause significant damage to the group dynamics. This person could be viewed as unreliable and lacking personal work ethics. If this person does not stand for some level of structured agreements within the group setting, he or she can quickly be viewed as inconsistent and a liability to the group.

As you can attest from the previous readings, there is no preferred method for group interactions that can ensure a successful outcome for a group. Instead, the preference is that all group members can recognize the preferences, validity, and contributions of each member. An individual can be highly competent and successful in academics or work, but just as every individual has significant strengths, everyone also has weaknesses. Whether your weakness is that you are highly analytical but cannot tie all the information together into a cohesive presentation, or that you are so highly structured in your time that you disregard the needs of the other group members, recognizing these needs in yourself can help you identify these strengths in others.

LESSON 2: RECOGNIZING THE PREFERENCES OF OTHERS

As a person with ASD, it is vital for you to develop an understanding about how teamwork can meet your needs. Instead of seeing the opportunity of working with people on projects as an anxiety-ridden experience, you can examine the strengths and preferences of others to build your team as you see fit. An effective team is made up of people with complementary strengths and preferences. A team that is made up of people with the same preferences and approaches to work could be positive and successful, but it is more likely that the team that is purposely made up of members that can challenge each other and contribute from different perspectives will be a more successful team.

Now that you have practiced evaluating your own preferences as a part of a team, you can use that same method to evaluate the preferences of other people. By recognizing the preferences of other people, you can put the right people on your team. By building a team in a logical way, the team can be effective and productive while allowing for a positive experience for all members.

PREFERENCE ANALYSIS OF OTHERS

Now that you have analyzed your preferences in group projects, identify one person you have worked with in the past on a project and use the same tool to identify his/her preferences in each of these pairs. Choose the statement that best represents how you viewed the interaction with the person. Once you have identified a preference between each pair, tally the number of responses for each side and circle the tallies on the number line under each. Each preference area can be a spectrum that can shift depending on the task and the person with whom you are working.

EXTROVERTED VS. INTROVERTED

E	I
☐ Likes being around a lot of people	☐ Takes a lot of energy to be in large groups
☐ Likes having many acquaintances	☐ Would rather have a few very close friends
☐ Can start a conversation with anyone	☐ Finds it hard to join a conversation
☐ Gets energy from being around people	☐ Gets energy from being alone and quiet
☐ Would rather be with a group of people than alone	☐ Would rather be alone or with a small group
☐ Enjoys parties and social events	☐ Enjoys movies or small group dinner parties
☐ Focused on what happens around them	☐ Focused on what happens within him/herself
☐ Tends to get bored easily when alone	☐ Tends to reflect and recharge when alone
☐ Tends to get revitalized and recharged when with others	☐ Tends to get overwhelmed and tired when with groups
☐ Has been described as enthusiastic or talkative	☐ Has been described as reflective or quiet

← 10 9 8 7 6 5 4 3 2 1 0 1 2 3 4 5 6 7 8 9 10 →

PRESENT VS. FUTURE

P	F
☐ Thinks about the current needs	☐ Often thinks about the end result
☐ Is concerned about meeting short-term goals	☐ Is concerned with meeting the large goal
☐ Wants to be able to complete a task today	☐ Can work on tasks over long periods of time
☐ Uses daily task lists	☐ Uses monthly/semester planning calendars
☐ Feels accomplishment when completing daily goals	☐ Feels accomplishment when planning strategically
☐ Waits until just before deadlines to start work	☐ Works on long-term projects in defined timelines
☐ Tends to overlook long-term projects	☐ Focuses heavily on meeting long-term project goals
☐ Can be described as a task completer	☐ Can be described as a planner
☐ Enjoys completing projects	☐ Enjoys planning projects
☐ Has been described as an activator	☐ Has been described as a planner

10 9 8 7 6 5 4 3 2 1 0 1 2 3 4 5 6 7 8 9 10

ANALYTICAL VS. CONTEXTUAL

A	C
☐ Feels comfortable finding results	☐ Feels comfortable making connections
☐ Likes working with data	☐ Likes organizing findings
☐ Is good working in groups with structure and routine	☐ Good working in groups that are free thinking and open
☐ Makes decisions based on results	☐ Makes decisions based on relating information
☐ Strength is in observing details	☐ Strength is in communicating results
☐ Would rather compile statistics	☐ Would rather present results
☐ Learn by doing analysis	☐ Learns by discussing results
☐ Tends to isolate details in problems	☐ Tends to look for linkages in solutions
☐ Can be described as a systemizer	☐ Can be described as a relator
☐ Likes working with mathematical equations	☐ Likes writing and presenting about results

10 9 8 7 6 5 4 3 2 1 0 1 2 3 4 5 6 7 8 9 10

STRUCTURED VS. FLEXIBLE

S	F
☐ Thinks that it is important to be on time	☐ Is usually on time
☐ Likes having detailed schedules to follow	☐ Typically work best with an open schedule
☐ Is comfortable with defined roles and duties	☐ Is comfortable with flexible role definitions
☐ Likes due dates and timelines	☐ Finds that due dates make things stressful
☐ Is comfortable when everyone stays on task	☐ Enjoys co-operative sharing of ideas
☐ Gets anxious when schedules are disrupted	☐ Can easily adjust to changes in schedules
☐ Thinks that if people are late it is disrespectful	☐ Thinks that it doesn't matter if people are late
☐ Enjoys working in a controlled environment	☐ Likes an environment where change is frequent
☐ Can be described as systematized	☐ Can be described as adaptable
☐ Would rather be in control of a project	☐ Would rather work in a collaborative group on a project

← →

10 9 8 7 6 5 4 3 2 1 0 1 2 3 4 5 6 7 8 9 10

LESSON 3: PARTNERING PREFERENCES TO BUILD TEAMS

Now that you have established the preferences of another person, compare how compatible your preferences are in each area. The intention of building a team in a logical way is to partner with people who have strengths and preferences that are different from your own. Analyze the strength of preference for yourself and the other person and reflect on how effective your partnership could be. Document the letter identifying the preference as well as the number identifying the strength (e.g. E3).

EXTROVERTED VS. INTROVERTED

Your preference

____

Other person's preference

____

What is the benefit of partnering with this person on a team?

____

____

____

____

____

____

____

What could be the potential pitfall if you are polar opposites?

____

____

____

____

____

____

____

____

PRESENT VS. FUTURE

Your preference

Other person's preference

What is the benefit of partnering with this person on a team?

What could be the potential pitfall if you are polar opposites?

ANALYTICAL VS. CONTEXTUAL

Your preference

____

Other person's preference

____

What is the benefit of partnering with this person on a team?

____

____

____

____

____

____

____

____

____

____

What could be the potential pitfall if you are polar opposites?

____

____

____

____

____

____

____

____

____

____

____

STRUCTURED VS. FLEXIBLE

Your preference

Other person's preference

What is the benefit of partnering with this person on a team?

What could be the potential pitfall if you are polar opposites?

LESSON 4: ROLES IN WORK TEAMS/GROUPS

The ability to analyze the preferences of other members of a team can also be beneficial as the team members begin to take on roles and responsibilities. Every member of a work team has something to contribute and recognizing the strengths and preferences can help frame the designation of the team roles and duties. Work teams typically are made up of roles that carry various responsibilities. As an example, four distinct roles will be introduced. These basic roles are typically represented on teams and it is safe to assume that most work groups will also include these roles among others. The four roles to be addressed in this activity are the motivator, the analyzer, the harmonizer, and the taskmaster. The preferences of the people who take on these roles can be evident in their role adoption. The preference combinations among people in these roles are not guaranteed, but can often be an indicator for what role the team member will choose. In the following activity, each role and potential preference combination will be presented. Take time to reflect on each description and identify the role you would adopt according to your personal preferences.

THE MOTIVATOR

The person in this role is typically the member who energizes the group to start the task at hand. He or she often takes a positive approach and focuses team conversations on the successful completion of the project. This person also recognizes when the team is losing energy and focus and can re-engage their focus on the end result. Finally, the role of motivator tends to be an action-focused role in which the person encourages ongoing participation and co-operation. The typical preference combination for this role is EFCF (Extroverted, Future, Contextual, Flexible).

THE ANALYZER

The person in this role is the member who focuses on the details of the project. The details that may seem unimportant to other members are vital to the person in this role. Each detail has an impact on the completion of the final product. This person can spend hours examining data, producing statistical findings, or researching information to support the group's work. The role of the analyzer tends to be a thought-focused role in which the person expels cognitive energy to ensure that the group presents the correct information. The typical preference combination for this role is IPAS (Introverted, Present, Analytical, Structured).

THE HARMONIZER

The person in this role tends to be highly focused on the equal participation of every member and often tries to make sure that each member feels heard and validated. The harmonizer tends to focus on the emotional energy of the group and find solutions when members are in conflict. This person often encourages the co-operation and communication process of the team as the members progress towards the goal. The role of harmonizer tends to be a person-focused role in which the person monitors the relationships and emotional stability of the team. The typical preference combination for this role is EPCF (Extroverted, Present, Contextual, Flexible).

THE TASKMASTER

The person in this role tends to be organized and focused on the assignment and completion of tasks by each member. The taskmaster sets timelines and goals for each team member and keeps the team focused on completing the goals by the established deadlines. The taskmaster seeks to avoid distractions and encourages team members to get their individual tasks completed so the team can meet their overall deadlines. The role of taskmaster tends to be an action-focused role in which the person focuses only on the objective work of each team member. The typical preference combination for this role is E-IPAS (Extroverted/Introverted, Present, Analytical, Structured).

Reflect on the descriptors associated with each of the team roles. Pay attention to the typical preference combination associated with each role as well. These preference combinations are typical, but not a rule. It is possible that your preference combination is not reflected in these roles. This does not mean that you do not have a role, it simply means that you may need to adjust how the role is defined on your team. With this information in mind, identify the role you could take on in a team that would make use of your strengths and preferences to help you successfully navigate a team project. In addition, identify the role that could be adopted by the other person you evaluated for preferences.

The difficulties that exist when a person is required to work as a part of a team can be amplified if the person is also a person with ASD. However, that is not to say that this task can not be done in a successful way. Many of the projects that are assigned in college or work have a co-operative component required to successfully complete the project. This requirement is not intended to make things more difficult for people with ASD, but is intended to encourage people to develop good work habits in preparation for careers. By working with others who have complementary strengths, you increase the likelihood that you will produce high-quality results. It is illogical to think that you will never have to work on a team, nor should you attempt to create ways to avoid working on teams. While it may be difficult to manage initially, and you may have to put in more effort to navigate the social requirements of the group, the benefits of completing a project with a team are tremendous.

Use the tools discussed in this chapter to analyze the preferences of not only yourself, but also the other members of your team. Identify the strengths or preferences of each member and build your team accordingly. Take a logical approach to analyzing the data and decide on role assignments based on this. Keep in mind that not all members will have the same working knowledge of preferences and roles in a team, but this can be a way to start the conversation about how the team intends to complete the task at hand. This should not be a license to take control of the group, but a way to assist the formation of an effective group that can be successful and have positive results for each member.

Reflect on your gained knowledge in this area and evaluate yourself honestly using the following BASICS chart.

BACK TO BASICS

Consider these guiding questions as you prepare to evaluate yourself.

B	**Behavior**	Do you recognize the preferences of people around you? Are you confident in demonstrating your own preferences? Are you communicating well in your group? Do you actively participate in a defined role in groups? Are you building teams that are effective in group tasks?
A	**Academics**	Are you attending all your classes on time? Are you applying organizational strategies? Are you consistently using your organizational system? Are you keeping up with everything?
S	**Self-care**	Are you getting enough sleep? Are you eating healthily? Are you planning for your self-care activities? Are you keeping your space clean? What are you doing to make sure you are managing your stress level?
I	**Interaction**	Are you checking in with your support team? Are you planning time for social activities? Are you actively engaged in classes? What are you doing to get to know your roommates? Are you checking your email/blackboard daily?
C	**Community**	Do you feel like you belong? Are you asking for help when needed? Have you met anyone new? Do you know the names of any classmates? Are you involved in anything socially?
S	**Self-monitoring**	Are you managing your time? Are you accepting critical feedback? Are you managing your frustration level? Are you willing to see the perspectives of others? Are you advocating for yourself?

BACK TO BASICS: RATE YOURSELF

B	**Behavior** 1 2 3	**Comments**
A	**Academics** 1 2 3	**Comments**
S	**Self-care** 1 2 3	**Comments**
I	**Interaction** 1 2 3	**Comments**
C	**Community** 1 2 3	**Comments**
S	**Self-monitoring** 1 2 3	**Comments**

GOALS

Personal:

Academic:

Social:

Chapter 8

CHANGING THE GOAL

Life is more than just earning a degree.

INTRODUCTION

Young adults with ASD can not only utilize knowledge of their own strengths and awareness of hidden social rules as they navigate college, but also as they begin to shift their focus to post-graduation employment. Changing the goal from academic success to career preparation can be a difficult process for neurotypicals and people with ASD alike. Students who have ASD might find the transition particularly challenging, but thinking about this transition earlier in their college career rather than later will help ease the shift in focus when it is actually time to apply for jobs.

Typically, students in their first one or two years of college are focusing on core classes, figuring out the social environment, and maintaining a satisfactory grade point average. This means that in the later semesters or years of college students will build on this social and academic foundation as the goal changes. At some point, young adults with ASD have to think about the next step after college. The next step will look different for every student. Some students will enter graduate level courses to pursue higher degrees, other students will take some time off to work on essential life skills, while others pursue employment immediately. Whatever the next step is, young adults need to know where they stand academically in the pursuit of graduation before decisions can be made about the future. Once the logistics of the present are considered, students can begin taking action toward their career goals.

For some young adults with ASD, standard and structured processes like the Career Continuum (see Lesson 3 on page 175) will provide guidance. Understanding the components of the Career Continuum, including community services, supervised and major internships and, finally, a career, will help young adults to know which of the components is a good idea for them. Students will also need to choose a major that actually fits their interests and goals. Then, learning the differences in and responsibilities of community service work, internships, and job shadowing can help students take effective steps toward building a marketable résumé. Lastly, knowing the role of a mentor and the dynamic of a mentoring relationship can make the other career steps much easier to understand and increase the chances that students follow through with those steps.

Access to a variety of potential workplace experiences and environments is essential for students on the spectrum who intend to enter a career upon graduating college. Consider showing up for the first day at a new job at an insurance company after college without having ever been in an office setting. The exposed cubicles and the process of "clocking in and out" or noting time of arrival and departure each day might be completely foreign to you. It would be like arriving on your college campus for the first time at 7:55 am for a class beginning at 8:00 am. Without an orientation to the campus, you would not know where to go or what to expect. This chapter encourages you to work through your options to assess potential opportunities even as a busy college student. Work through the lessons to determine where you are currently in the career process and consider how to use your college resources to create a marketable résumé while earning your degree at the same time.

LESSON 1: LOOKING FORWARD

Creating a realistic plan from an abstract notion of future career goals for the next two to six years can be a challenging endeavor for many young adults, especially those who have ASD. In order to actively work toward career goals, you must create some kind of realistic plan with concrete steps and achievable goals. The first step involves one of the most important factors worth exploring as you prepare for major life transitions like life after college, which is knowing the state of your current situation. It is a lot like solving a puzzle. First, you need to know what you have to work with before you can make the next move. As a college student, you need to be aware of some logistics of your situation. It can be quite easy to be caught up in the social and academic pressures of any college semester, and that is especially true for those in the first few semesters at college. But establishing a solid understanding of where you stand in terms of graduation progress and career interests during these first few semesters can make a big difference in the way the rest of your college time progresses.

If you wait until the semester you are expected to graduate to find that you have missed several courses needed for your degree or that you have not added any experience to your résumé, it can create significant distracting stressors in an already stressful time. Thinking about things like minimal credit hours needed, core course completion requirements, mandatory grade point average for the college and your major, and potential internships and job shadowing placements as you go through the early semesters and throughout your time at college can make this transition much smoother. It will also help you establish yourself as a marketable future employee.

Young adults work with advisors, mentors, instructors, career and employment co-ordinators, and an array of other people to navigate the process of shifting focus from academic college work—the "here and now"—to the future, a career. The continuous process throughout college leading up to a career involves utilizing some of the social skills you read about and discussed in the previous chapter. You will also need to tailor your communication depending on who you are working with for any of the steps involved in your career plan. This is important to note because it is very unlikely that you will complete these steps without the guidance of other people on your campus who usually have special skills used specifically to help students through this process. While it is your future and ultimately your own decisions that are at the forefront of the discussions you will have with these supporting people, you have access to the input and insight of those who have been through the process before and have information about your particular field from which you will undoubtedly benefit. Essentially, know you are not alone in this process. College is a place for academic work and education, of course, but you are also probably paying for the supporting services that help make sure you can actually pursue your career goals with the knowledge you have learned in the classroom.

Take some time to contemplate the supporting people you might be able to work with throughout your time at college before you graduate. You can use the following table to record their details.

SUPPORTING OFFICES/ROLES	NAME	CONTACT INFORMATION	NOTES
EXAMPLE: Career and Student Employment Services	Marie Hurst	University Center, Room 300 656-010–3490 Marie.Hurst@univ.edu	• Career Fair in Spring Semester • Résumé workshops • Interview practice
Career and Student Employment Services			
Disability Resource Center			
Favorite Instructor in your Major Program			
Peer Groups/Student Organizations			
Professional Mentor			
Academic Advisor			

Now that you know who can help you through this process, it is a good idea to start thinking about how you are doing academically. As a college student, you are working toward completing all the courses necessary to receive a degree. A college degree is often a requirement for many careers, especially in those fields that are highly specialized. Maintaining at least the minimum grade point average necessary for graduation should be an obvious goal. Most internships and graduate school opportunities demand a grade point average well above the minimum, though. That means that you need to know what the minimum grade point average is for graduating with a college degree, but you also need to do some research to figure out what grade point average internships in your field require or what you would need to maintain for consideration as a graduate school candidate. You will probably also have a particular minimum grade point average for your major program that might be different from the overall university minimum and you might also have scholarship funds dependent on a certain grade point average.

What are the different grade point averages that you need to be aware of at your college and in your major program?

Goal	Minimum Grade Point Average
Remaining in "good standing" at your college	
Local internship in your field	
Graduate school admission	
Overall cumulative average	
Maintaining scholarships	

For students on the spectrum, intense special interests can be the driving force for a college degree and future career. In fact, many students thrive in the courses they take that are aligned with their interests despite significant challenges in the core curriculum courses that are often required as prerequisites for the more specialized upper-level courses. Not only must students take those general courses that might not directly apply to their field, but they must also do well enough in each of them to count as credit hours toward degree completion. For example, if your major is History, you might have to successfully take a certain number of English or composition courses before moving on to upper-level History courses. There is a benefit to having to take these courses, though. For many college students, these courses provide insight into fields previously not considered. It also is not unheard of for students to change their academic major after taking an introductory course in their program and finding that it is not actually what they had in mind for a career. Taking the first few semesters seriously, even when you might think you are not interested in some courses, will help you maintain a satisfactory grade point average and allow you to have the experience necessary to make decisions about your future.

LESSON 2: CHOOSING THE RIGHT ACADEMIC MAJOR

As a young adult with ASD, one of your strengths might be that you have a unique, intense interest in a particular subject. That is a definite asset in the challenge of deciding on an academic major. Choosing a major is one of the most important decisions you make while you are a college student. If you have already chosen your major, read through this lesson and evaluate your current major as if you were comparing it to another option. The benefit of choosing a major that is interesting to pursue academically through focused coursework is that you will have motivation to succeed academically and curiosity and interest to understand interesting material beyond the classroom, which may prompt you to seek out community service or a local internship. Some young adults with ASD may struggle with deciding how to focus their academic efforts and commit to taking action in the direction of a career. Fortunately, the pressure of choosing the right major can be alleviated with the knowledge that there is a significant population of students who end up working in a field unrelated to their academic major in college.

Declaring a major, though, establishes purpose and focus. When you select a major, you designate many hours of your coursework to a particular focused area. You will work with a set of professors and advisors who have knowledge and experience in your field of interest. The benefit of focus and purpose to your academic career at college is great, especially for students on the spectrum. Studying for a course that fits a particular interest area for you provides an outlet for interest-related strengths. Structure in the form of program checklists, knowledgeable advisors, interest-driven social interaction, templates for scheduling, and consistent instructor availability can be significant factors in a successful college experience. Choosing a major that is interesting to you ensures that you are more likely to commit to spending time and energy studying a particular subject, yielding positive academic results and readying you for work in a major-related career.

Narrowing down your options for a major can be difficult, but you can compare some key aspects of each potential program to help you make an informed decision. In Figure 8.2, compare two or more possible majors that interest you. Fill in the chart with important factors you need to consider if you are deciding between a few options for your major. Consider how each of the elements impacts you and your learning needs. See the example in Figure 8.1 if you need a prompt.

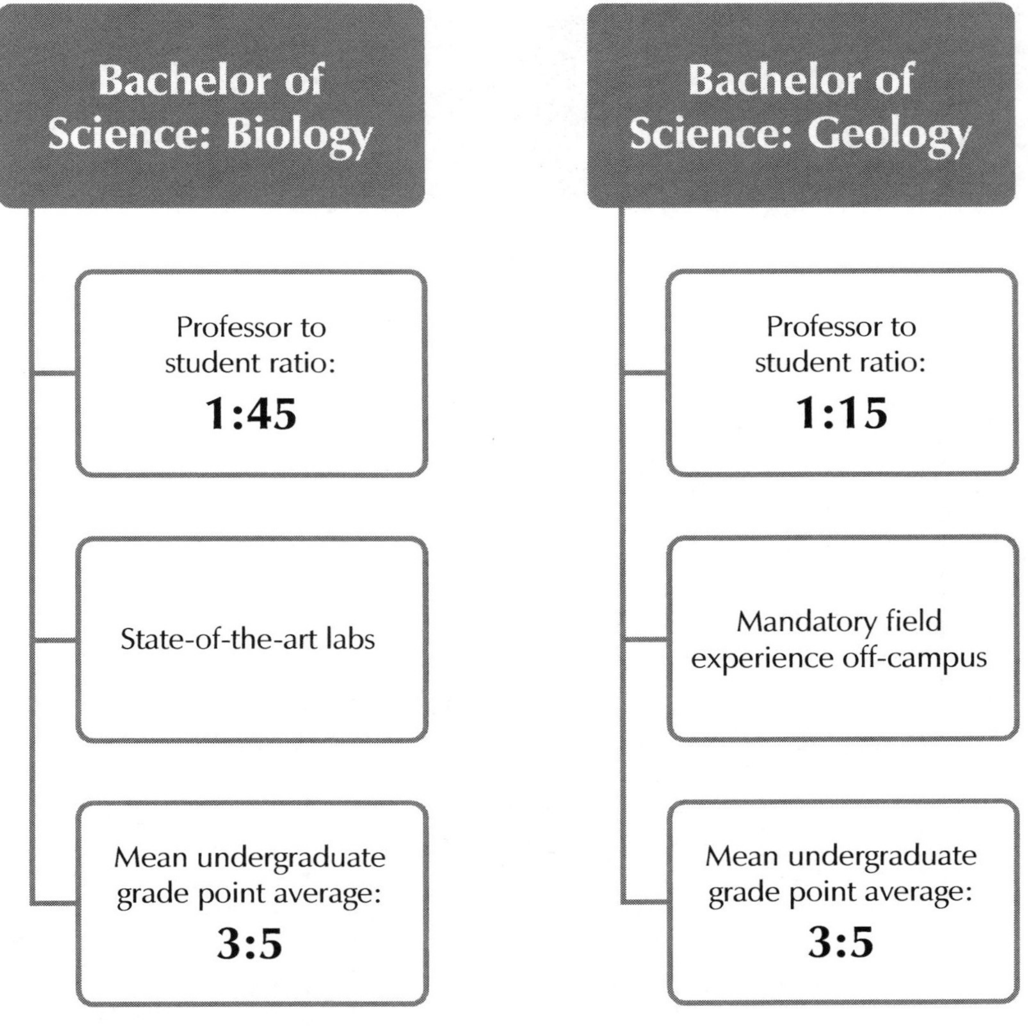

FIGURE 8.1: ACADEMIC MAJOR COMPARISON (EXAMPLE)

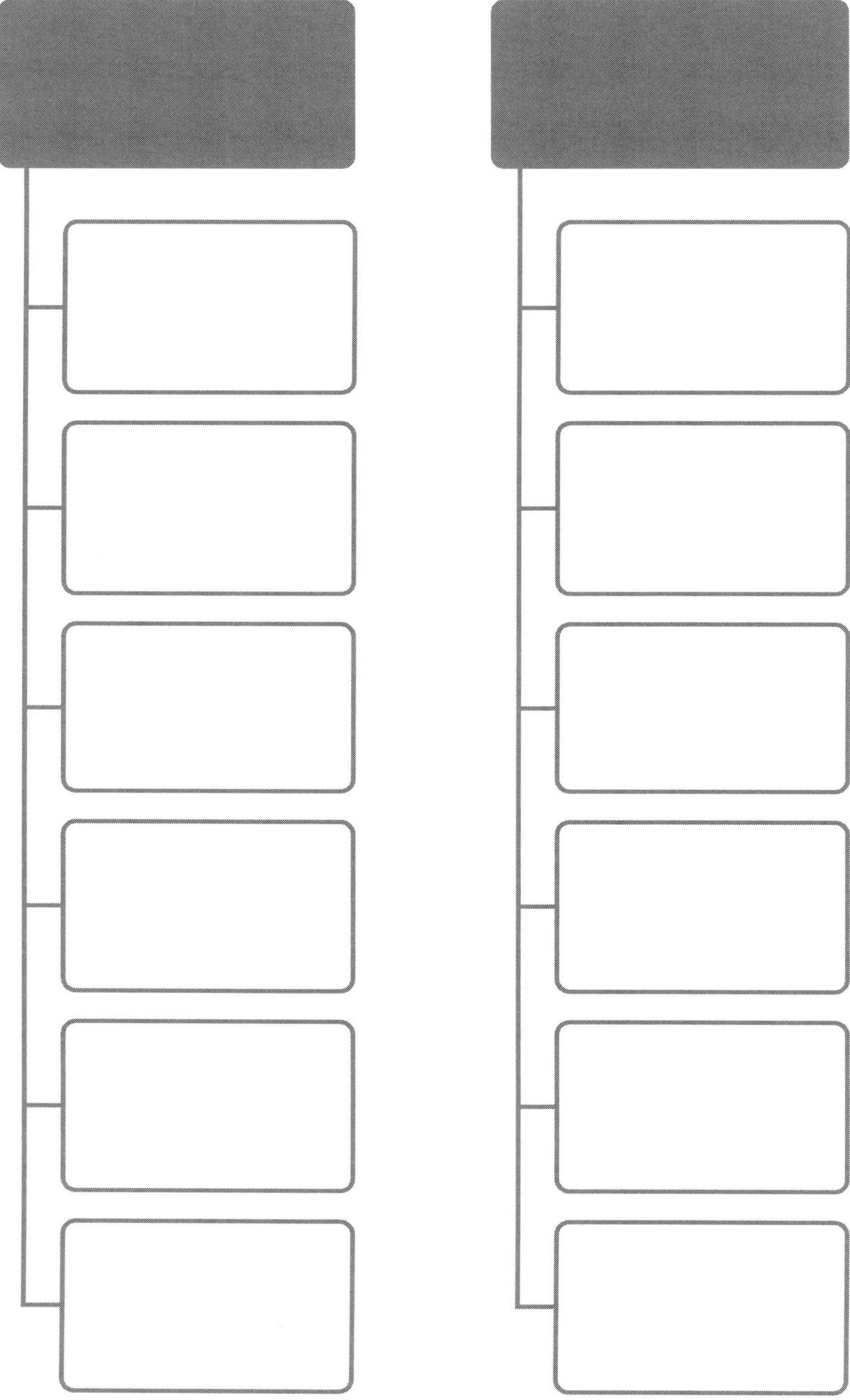

FIGURE 8.2: ACADEMIC MAJOR COMPARISON

LESSON 3: THE CAREER CONTINUUM

There are a few characteristics of the process of planning for your future while in college that many successful students utilize to move forward intentionally. As students build their experience beyond the classroom, they have the opportunity to further strengthen pre-existing interests or to realize new interests. While there is not one complete set of steps that would apply to every situation, there are at least four components of this process, which combined we call the Career Continuum. The four components are community service, supervised internships, major internships, and, lastly, a career. They will be discussed in order from community service to career since these elements in this model are progressive, building experience and responsibility with each of the four components.

Examine Figure 8.3 and reflect on the experiences you have had in each of the four distinct areas. If you have not yet developed a continuum to enter your career, you may use this visual as a way to direct your experiences.

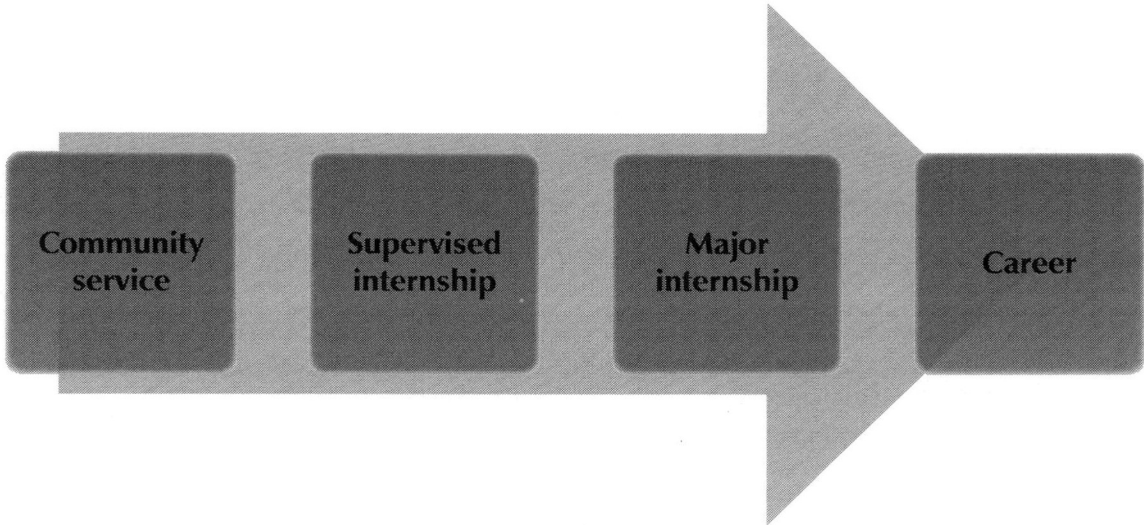

FIGURE 8.3: CAREER CONTINUUM

DEFINED STEPS

1. COMMUNITY SERVICE

Community service is working, often voluntarily, to strengthen an aspect of your immediate community. You might have been required to fulfill some community service portion of a high school course in your home town. If you have relocated for college, community service is something you may take part in your college town or in your hometown during holidays or breaks. Sometimes community service is directly related to your interest area, but working in your community in any element is a good way to demonstrate to future employers that you value the community in which you may one day earn a living. College is a great space to explore community service options.

2. SUPERVISED INTERNSHIPS

Supervised internships provide you with direct access to learn the environment in which you could work should you decide to pursue a career in the field. These internships will probably be in your chosen career field or one of a few serious fields of interest. A supervised internship in each of a few of your options could help you determine the best kind of work environment for you and your goals. As an intern at this level, you will have limited responsibilities and work directly with a mentor who provides you with guidance navigating the new environment. Supervised internships, which are typically short-term, serve to show you the culture of a workplace and allow you to begin thinking about what kind of accommodations you might need if you were to work in a workplace that is arranged in a similar manner.

3. MAJOR INTERNSHIPS

A major internship is one that is directly related to your academic major and career goals. Major internships allow you to experience an authentic and, often intensive, interview process. Candidates at this level are generally chosen from a competitive selection of applicants. Interns at this level have real responsibility and such internships serve as a real opportunity to turn a positive and productive internship experience into a full-time career with the same or a similar company. Your role as an intern will also prompt your development of job-related self-advocacy skills, which may include disclosing ASD and requesting accommodations.

4. CAREER

A career is a full-time, interest-driven professional occupation. As an employee, you are likely to earn a salary and consistent income. Careers can be long-term endeavors. You will have position or role-specific duties and responsibilities. If you perform well, there is potential for promotion and advancement within a company or field. In many cases, employees gain experience leading to leadership positions, such as management roles. In your career, you will have many professional development opportunities, such as research visits to other similar work sites, professional conferences, workshops, webinars, and job-related training.

Fill in the following chart with your ideas about each of the four components. Be sure to write down any experience you have currently in any of the four areas, or write down possible ideas to pursue in one or all categories.

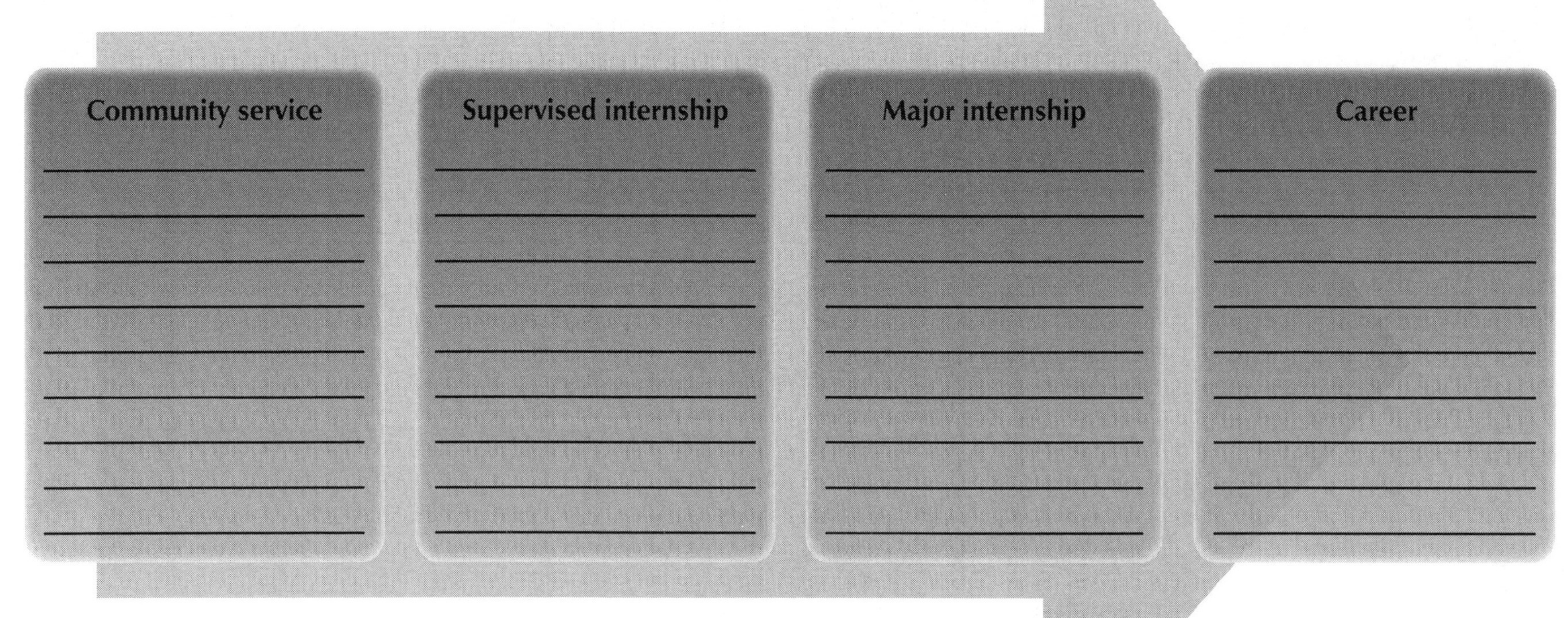

Figure 8.4: Your Career Continuum

CREATE YOUR OWN PATH

It is important to remember that while the Career Continuum provides some structure to the process of navigating your job search, there is certainly a chance that your own process might look quite different. The Career Continuum that we have provided is a general outline with proven steps, but these steps might be rearranged to fit your goals and your timeline. You might even miss a component entirely. Some students on the spectrum choose to spend some time after college working on life skills, like learning how to drive or learning independent living skills. Other students network well and incidentally create opportunities for an entry-level job in a field that fits their interests before ever having completed any community service. Your experience will be unique. You will adapt to your own circumstances and goals and your path will reflect that.

Take some time to think about some elements you think your path will include. These can include the four components we outlined in the Career Continuum, but you will also need to consider any other potential future pieces to include in your own path. Do you intend to pursue a Master's or Doctorate degree? What life skills will you need to master before living independently and working full-time? Do you intend to work a part-time job during your time at college? Think about these questions and any other factors you might experience in the next few years as you go through college. Write those factors and any relevant details in the table below.

Factor in Creating Your Own Path	Relevant Planning Details
Example: Master's degree in Anthropology	Two years of intensive courses Field experience required

Now that you know how your own path might differ from the Career Continuum and the limits of the four components, work out a potential timeline or general trajectory for these factors leading up to a career that interests you. Use the example to guide your own visual representation.

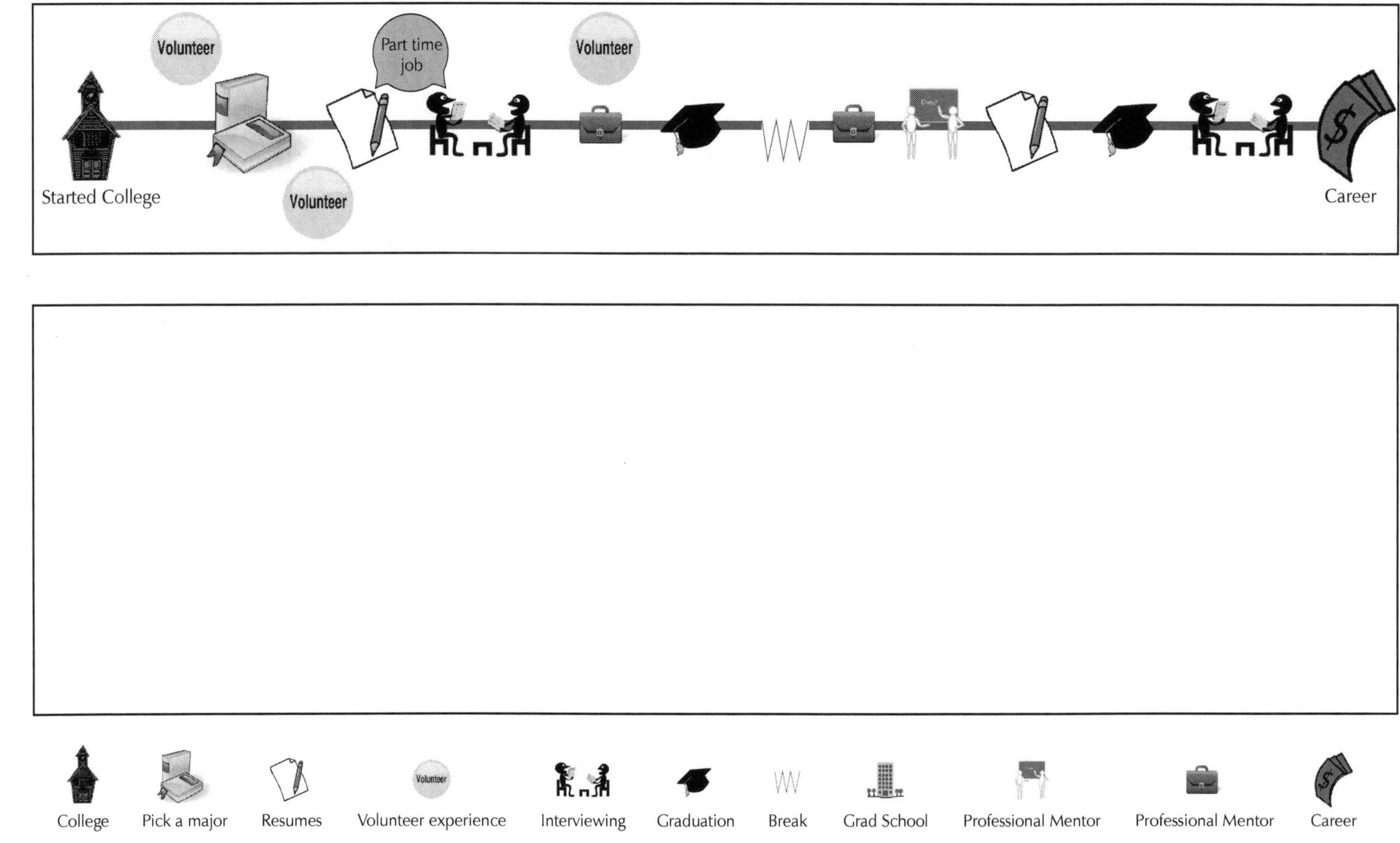

LESSON 4: AN INTRODUCTION TO COMMUNITY SERVICE, JOB SHADOWING, AND INTERNSHIPS

Examining the progression of the Career Continuum and the process of outlining your own possible path can help you gather some ideas for building career-relevant experience into your time as a college student. As a student with ASD, it is important that you have a chance to explore many environments to help you narrow down your career possibilities as you progress through completing your college degree. You have access to a supportive network of professionals, a catalog of fascinating courses, and experts in your interest area standing at the front of your lecture hall. The setting is perfect for pursuing interests and gaining valuable experience before beginning a full-time career. Three common "stepping stones" on many paths to a career for college students are involvement in community service, gathering on-site observation time, and serving as an intern to learn the intricate workings of a certain work environment or field.

COMMUNITY SERVICE

There is an abundance of community service opportunities on college campuses. Campus organizations, religious groups, academic clubs, fraternities and sororities, and honor societies are some of the groups tied to your college environment that are likely to foster community service opportunity. Some of these groups even require a set number of hours spent serving the community in some way to maintain membership. For example, some honor societies have partnerships with community members who serve to connect campus to a need in the community. In order to maintain status in the elite group of students who adhere to a high level of academic standard, members of an academic honors-based club with this requirement will not only be strong employment candidates because of academic success, but also because of a demonstration of serving the community. The relationship between your effort in serving the community and its benefit can be described as one that is symbiotic. In this case, specifically, your community is strengthened through your actions and service to make it better and your career potential increases with your experience of helping others.

JOB SHADOWING

Spending time in the environment of a potential workplace and observing an employee acting in a role that interests you is a great way to simply take in the information you can from the setting. You will have a chance to watch, assessing the environment and structure of the activity in the workplace, staff peer-to-peer interactions, and sensory stimuli. A career counselor at your college can point you to local professionals in your field and can help you construct an appropriate script for requesting to shadow an employee. College instructors, academic advisors, and program department administration are also useful resources in identifying possible job shadowing opportunities. When you are job shadowing, you are merely observing and you will not have any responsibilities, unlike internships. Keep in mind that job shadowing is typically a one-day event, but it may be arranged for you to observe regularly.

INTERNSHIPS

Internships are designed to allow interested people the chance to learn about the field in a real setting. Interns can do a wide variety of tasks with a range of responsibility. Internships are essentially a platform for gaining work-related experience in a structured setting. Companies or businesses that hire interns often view this as a form of inexpensive and valuable service. They may be short or long-term, typically term-based, like during the summer or throughout one academic semester. In some cases, you may receive college credit for your internship. Your instructors, advisors, and career counselors are resources for you as you seek out local internship applications.

Differentiating internships for job shadowing and community service is the interview and selection process. Internships are regarded highly among college students and a large pool of interested people to choose from means that internship selection may be competitive. Maintaining a strong grade point average and interpersonal relationship with professional contacts that you can network with for potential internship opportunities can help you to stand out among applicants. When considering an internship, do not ignore logistical factors like flexibility in scheduling since you are still a college student with deadlines and class meetings. Use the following short exercise to brainstorm ideas relating to community service, job shadowing, and internships. Things to consider include any current relevant contacts who can help point you to one of these "stepping stones," whether or not you are a member of any organizations with a structured arrangement for community service, if you are academically prepared for the increased responsibility you will have with an internship, and whatever other important aspect you need to consider.

Under each category, brainstorm potential contacts or companies with whom you can make contact so you can work through your Career Continuum.

Community Service

Job Shadowing

Internships

LESSON 5: MENTORS AND CAREER PREPARATION

Having a person you trust to help you navigate the Career Continuum and job preparation process while you are in college can make a significant difference. Students with ASD can benefit from a mentor while they are in college. A mentor has a multifaceted role. He or she can provide accountability, structure, recognition and utilization of your individual strengths as someone who has ASD, valuable insight into the student's field of interest, and career preparation strategies. This lesson will explore the many benefits of working with a mentor during college and, finally, you will discuss some general strategies for career preparation while you are in college and how a mentor can help.

UNDERSTANDING MENTORS

The relationship between a mentor and you is professional and should be regarded as such. That is not to say that your relationship with your mentor would not be authentic. In fact, establishing boundaries and guidelines for the interactions can help you quickly develop a routine and lessen the chances of social confusion. Setting up the relationship does not have to be a formal process. Essentially, you can set up consistency in the first few meetings with a mentor. Work with your mentor to create a checklist of topics to cover each time you meet. You might check in once a month to review possible job shadowing contacts or community service opportunities. These occasional topics might include scripting a request for information at a career fair at your college or a demonstration of how to navigate your college's career center website to look for volunteer placements. You should also decide on the logistical arrangements, like how often you will meet and where, or clarifying through which mode you will communicate between appointments. These might not be issues that you need to firmly establish, but be respectful of your mentor's time by being consistent. Working with a mentor throughout any period of college, no matter how long, teaches you skills and resourcefulness that will certainly aid you during your career preparation.

There are a number of characteristics you will need to seek out in a potential mentor. When you consider the nature of the relationship, you might think of characteristics like honesty and compassion, which allow truthful insights to be shared in a safe space. You should feel comfortable practicing social interactions with your mentor, as he or she will be helping you practice for interviews, for example, and explaining workplace social context when necessary. Another important aspect of a mentor to consider is personality. You should work with someone with whom you genuinely like to work. There may be certain specific characteristics you will look for in a potential mentor.

What comes to mind when you think of an ideal mentor?

CAREER PREPARATION

Young adults in college can utilize some strategies for preparing for their career while they are still taking classes and keeping busy with extra-curricular and social events. While you may be many semesters away from applying for your first "real job," it is not too early to start working on building your résumé and learning how to interview well. This career preparation process, if you were to cram it into a single semester before you graduate college, could be rather similar to a job in terms of time commitment. Avoid the added stress of this process in those final semesters by committing to a few career preparation strategies early in your college career to give you a leading start.

One strategy that is worth exploring early on in your college career is developing and building your résumé. A résumé is a summative document that reflects your primary objectives in applying for jobs and the skills and experience that qualify you for jobs. Your résumé will include your contact information, your education experience, your previous work history, reference contact information, and your most marketable awards, memberships, skills, and talents. This document holds quite a bit of weight for you during the application process for jobs. The résumé is all a potential employer might have to compare your experience with that of others applying for the same job. Spend time during college engaging in organizations, clubs, honors societies, and community service to build the information you can put on your résumé.

Another career preparation strategy you might consider is engaging in structured practice interviews. For internships, exclusive honors societies, and jobs, the interview can be one of the most important elements of the application process. Interviews allow potential employers to meet you, ask direct questions about your experience, establish the reason you are interested in a job, and also allow you to seek information from the interviewer. Here, perhaps with more significance than other social interactions, making a good first impression is essential. You will need to enter an interview meeting with confidence and be able to project this confidence well. You will be assessed not only for your skills and experience, but also for your ability to work with other people. There are several ways to improve your interviewing skills, but one of the most effective ways is simply to practice. You can work with your mentor or the career services center on your campus for practice interviews. You will have a chance to receive direct feedback on your interview performance each time, so you will know how to improve as you keep practicing for future real interviews. Remember to treat these as if they are real interviews by dressing appropriately and arriving on time.

Taking the time to prepare a résumé and to practice interviewing is an important way for you to prepare for future employment. Receiving feedback on your strengths and weaknesses in interviews can make you more prepared to enter a real interview with the confidence you will need to show the employer you are a good candidate for a position. When you practice, you might find that you need to work on making eye contact or that you need to rethink your interview outfit. For students with ASD, preparing for these key career elements like your résumé and interview can make the actual process of applying for jobs and interviewing for them more familiar and less overwhelming.

As you prepare to move to the next phase in your education and career, evaluate yourself on your gained knowledge. Use the following BASICS chart to honestly rate your growth.

BACK TO BASICS

Consider these guiding questions as you prepare to evaluate yourself.

B	**Behavior**	What are you doing to keep track of your grade point average? Are you regularly checking in with your academic advisor? Are you succeeding in courses in your academic major? Are you actively seeking community service, job shadowing, and internship options? Are you regularly meeting with a mentor for career preparation?
A	**Academics**	Are you attending all your classes on time? Are you applying organizational strategies? Are you consistently using your organizational system? Are you keeping up with everything?
S	**Self-care**	Are you getting enough sleep? Are you eating healthily? Are you planning for your self-care activities? Are you keeping your space clean? What are you doing to make sure you are managing your stress level?
I	**Interaction**	Are you checking in with your support team? Are you planning time for social activities? Are you actively engaged in classes? What are you doing to get to know your roommates? Are you checking your email/blackboard daily?
C	**Community**	Do you feel like you belong? Are you asking for help when needed? Have you met anyone new? Do you know the names of any classmates? Are you involved in anything socially?
S	**Self-monitoring**	Are you managing your time? Are you accepting critical feedback? Are you managing your frustration level? Are you willing to see the perspectives of others? Are you advocating for yourself?

BACK TO BASICS: RATE YOURSELF

B	**Behavior** 1 2 3	**Comments**
A	**Academics** 1 2 3	**Comments**
S	**Self-care** 1 2 3	**Comments**
I	**Interaction** 1 2 3	**Comments**
C	**Community** 1 2 3	**Comments**
S	**Self-monitoring** 1 2 3	**Comments**

GOALS

Personal:

Academic:

Social:

NEXT STEPS

Students with ASD in college experience significant personal growth. When their perceptions and strengths are aligned to result in positive outcomes, their experience with personal growth will help them prepare for the next steps. Transitioning focus from learning how college students can navigate the academic and social demands to a focus that is interest-driven and career-oriented can be a challenging process for many students. With the right tools and strategies, however, students will approach the career preparation process with confidence and the skill necessary to be successful.

The next step of the BASICS curriculum is designed to foster career exploration. Students will engage actively with their own strengths and interests to take practical steps toward a career after college. Students with ASD will be guided through common steps in the career exploration process and develop skills and strategies to navigate the increasing social demands involved in intentional career planning. Relying on their strengths, students will complete the next curriculum with new knowledge of a career path that is interesting and realistic, all the while gaining valuable insight into their own potential contributions to their chosen field.

Appendix A

BASICS CHART STUDENT EXAMPLE

B	**Behavior** 1 2 **3**	**Comments** I am starting to become more aware of some of my behaviors. I really like when people offer me suggestions as long as I am sure what they mean by them. I am still working on identifying areas in which challenges are presented but I am more aware of areas that I am experiencing growth in.
A	**Academics** 1 **2** 3	**Comments** I am starting to really lean on my support team. I am attending all but my geology class because it is at 8 am and I cannot get out of bed. I still need to complete 2 of the 4 study hours.
S	**Self-care** 1 **2** 3	**Comments** I go to bed every night around 11 pm and get up around 8 am so I am getting enough sleep. My roommates have been complaining of my messy room so I probably need to clean it.
I	**Interaction** **1** 2 3	**Comments** I do not like speaking up in class or checking my email. I would much rather play a video game in my room or listen to music. I am not used to all these people constantly being around me.
C	**Community** 1 **2** 3	**Comments** Sometimes I feel like I am so different but when I am around others in this class I see there are people like me out there. I don't typically like meeting new people but most of us have common interests so that has been really cool.
S	**Self-monitoring** 1 **2** 3	**Comments** I realize now that I could do a better job advocating for myself so that is one of my new goals for the semester. I really am not good at time management but since I started using my phone for reminders I am getting better.

Appendix B

GUIDED DISCUSSION

In this section, points of discussion and guiding questions are offered for each chapter. This information is intended to be a starting point for conversation and should be built upon based on the needs of the group, class, or individual. These suggestions are proposed to provoke thought about the material, and it is the hope of the authors that each user will build upon these suggestions to make this material useful for each user.

CHAPTER 1: PERSONAL STORIES

LESSON 1: EARLY CHILDHOOD

Discussion Points

Everyone has a story to tell. These stories are a combination of unique experiences and some of your earliest childhood memories. For individuals diagnosed with ASD, some of the earliest memories could be centered on the challenges faced in early childhood. Inevitably, one's experiences shape how a person views oneself, or what we call self-perception. In a way it paves the way to adulthood. For most individuals on the autism spectrum it is likely that they experience things very differently from most neurotypicals, but these memories still impact self-perception. A way to explore how events contribute to shaping each student's self-perception is to ask that they explore some of these early childhood memories by creating a narrative or what is called a personal story in the text. By reflecting on these early memories one could gain insight as to why they react to things the way they do and how they sometimes view certain qualities. Sometimes these memories bring up difficult topics and strong emotions, but doing so allows the individuals opportunity and encouragement to move past the barriers of their past and reframe their negative views into more positive ones. Students will need to spend time exploring how their earliest memories impact how they view themselves and the memories they hold on to. Taking some time to recall these memories and experiences with likeminded people will give them a chance to move towards understanding one another. The impact can either be positive or negative, understood or misunderstood, and it is worth exploring through the personal stories of early childhood experiences.

Parents, teachers, doctors, and sometimes peers have been known to impact individuals in some way. In this section, we explore how they have impacted each one differently.

Guiding Questions

- How did people around you view you as a child?
- What are some details you remember about your childhood?
- What are a few important memories you have that made a lasting impression on you?
- What early childhood memories impacted your self-perception?
- Were there any discussions about your diagnosis or reactions that stand out to you from parents, teachers, or others?
- What things were difficult during your early childhood?

LESSON 2: TEEN YEARS

Discussion Points

Regardless of an ASD diagnosis, being a teenager in general can be a difficult experience. It is known for being a difficult time in one's life as one begins to navigate through the world of social norms. It is a time in one's life in which change is a common theme. Hormones are changing, social status seems vital, and understanding some of the new social norms can be some of the areas that will change during this time. For someone with ASD, this can be even harder and more confusing. Everyone is looking for where they fit in, dodging bullies, and struggling to feel like they belong in a group. During this time it is difficult to avoid negative messages when someone doesn't fit in to what they think they are supposed to. Social media makes this a much more difficult experience then it was years ago. It gives an outlet but if not managed appropriately it can have different uses. This is when bullying is at an all-time high and sometimes students get lost in comparing themselves to others. Recognizing that this is a time full of difficult transitions and a time when one's quirks may become more noticeable, students must reflect on what it was like for them because the experiences of one's teen years contribute significantly to one's self-perception. For students with ASD this might be a period of time in which they became more self-aware of their differences and faced feelings of isolation. By reflecting on their own personal experience during the teenage years they might gain a better understanding of some of the negative perceptions they have about themselves. Although some of the memories might be more positive than others, each memory plays a part in how they view themselves in their community, whether that be on a college campus, in a job, or in their personal life.

Guiding Questions

- What changed from your early childhood as you became a teenager?
- What social rules changed?
- How did you adjust?
- Were there times you felt bullied? If so, name a few.
- During your teenage years, did you ever feel isolated?
- What are some negative messages you heard and how has that impacted you today?
- What about positive messages?
- Did anyone ever complain about your behaviors?
- What were some difficult transitions for you during your teen years?

LESSON 3: YOUNG ADULTHOOD

Discussion Points

The transition to college is a time when individuals are challenged in a whole new way. Suddenly those things that made an individual stand out and defined identity are now blended into crowds so they do not feel as unique as they once did. Students may have been seen as the smartest one in their class, but in college everyone is smart. Individuals on the autism spectrum are capable of succeeding academically in college but often get held up when it comes to social experiences. One's early childhood memories in addition to teen experiences can have a huge impact on self-perception in adulthood. How students identify themselves in the context of their environment affects how they transition into these new stages of life. During this time students have a lot of choices to make, are exposed to new levels of responsibility, choose a major, learn how to effectively manage time, and work on learning more about themselves by exploring new things. Some of the changes they might experience during this time can be overwhelming and confusing. It is important for them to reflect on their personal stories from each period of their life to gain the insight needed to make the best out of this transition. By gaining this insight, students will learn to navigate the world around them, which here and now is on a college campus. During this time students might be experiencing a huge shift in relationships as they work on developing new friendships and even beginning to explore romantic relationships. How one enters both casual and romantic relationships is impacted by one's self-perceptions. Ultimately, this is the time in which students must become more future-minded.

Guiding Questions

- How did you react to the environment around you as a young adult?
- How did you handle transitions?
- What did or do you perceive to be new social rules during this time?
- Do you feel like you lost a part of your identity?
- How did your views of yourself change?
- What are some ways you can challenge yourself to think about things differently?
- Identify some important relationships around you.
- What are some changes you have made in your personal life?
- What level of respect do you have for yourself?

LESSON 4: WRITING YOUR OWN STORY

Discussion Points

Reflecting on developmental periods of one's life allows one to examine the impact that others have had on shaping who one is becoming. Some memories are more difficult than others and some do not play an active role in how individuals view their life today; also, some experiences will have been more positive than others. The important thing for individuals with ASD, in this case students, to remember about this part of their journey is that ultimately everyone has a unique experience and each story can be very difficult. Students are asked to write their own personal stories and, if possible, share what they feel comfortable with. The idea is to validate and somewhat normalize their experience with likeminded peers. Each experience for someone with ASD is very different but more often than not there are some common themes worth exploring.

Guiding Questions

- How does it feel to know you have power to write your story and change the outcome?
- What is it like for you to read or hear about similar experiences from your peers with ASD?
- Why is it important to understand what you want others to see in you?
- How have you grown and how can you view the future more positively?
- What have you changed about how you view yourself?
- What do you have control of?

CHAPTER 2: THE LANGUAGE OF ASD

LESSON 1: IDENTITY MODELS

Discussion Points

Neurodiversity, accounting for natural variations in the human brain, is a concept that can be explained through one of two models. College students can look at these two models, the diagnostic and identity models, to consider how language and labeling factors contribute to their notions of ASD. Students reflect on their own experiences with each model's characteristics, through identifying the goal, message, focus, language, identity, and processing for each. As students consider the differences in identity and diagnostic models, they can use their knowledge to serve as a lens through which they will learn to view ASD.

Guiding Questions

- What experiences contribute to your view of ASD in each model?
- Which of the characteristics of the model do you have a strong reaction to?
- What is neurodiversity?
- How does language impact these identity models?

LESSON 2: DIAGNOSTIC LANGUAGE

Discussion Points

In recent years, there has been a huge push to promote diversity on college campuses. This push emphasizes ideas such as student identity and awareness. Diversity will enhance the college experience for all. This is a time in students' lives when they are developing their identity. Maybe this is the first time a student is having to independently work through anything related to their disability. Neurodiversity is a term that suggests that differences in the human brain can be attributed simply to natural variation. In a sense, it embraces differences of various disability and diversity groups, including autism spectrum disorders, as having distinctive characteristics, rather than being seen as broken or needing to be fixed. Typically, when someone starts talking about diagnostic language there is some kind of connection made with stereotyping and labels that have been recognized as the negative stuff we have mentioned in previous chapters. Although this might be a difficult process for some individuals, the purpose is to highlight the level of impact ASD has had on an individual and to provide an opportunity for a more positive discussion about the so-called deficits with likeminded peers. By having these discussions in a trusting environment with individuals with similar experience, the hope is that students will begin to normalize their negative views and make the shift to having a positive outlook of the impact of ASD. It has been proven through various studies and student-led discussions that this diagnostic process was an experience that significantly impacted their self-perceptions. Being open and honest will help students see the impact and make the shift to a more positive, but realistic, perception of the individual.

Guiding Questions

- What parts of diagnostic language stand out to you?
- How has diagnostic language impacted how you view yourself as someone on the spectrum?
- What level of impact did this process have on you?
- What strategies have you started or could you start developing to see the diagnosis as something positive?

LESSON 3: IDENTITY LANGUAGE

Discussion Points

There is a vast difference between diagnostic language and identity language discussed in this chapter. Throughout the course of one's life, people, experiences, and environment impact how we view the world around us but also how we view ourselves. So often young adults get caught up worrying about what others think or have said about them and that is how they define their identity. Identity is not defined through the eyes of others, which is an important point to address with students with ASD. It is time for them to start reflecting on their own experiences and what makes them unique. The great thing about college is that students are allowed the opportunity to gain exposure to a diverse setting and differing populations of people in a safe environment. To have new experiences that begin to shape and redefine one's identity is significant to individuals set on reaching their full potential. For individuals with ASD, this might be a time when they begin to positively identify with the diagnosis and how they associate with ASD. The identity criterion was developed to help alleviate negative emotions or stigmas and gain a more positive perspective/insight to the diagnosis. This will help students identify their potential and reframe some of their negative perceptions into more positive ones.

Guding Questions

- What experiences helped shape you?
- What interest and characteristics shape how you define yourself?
- What titles have stuck with you throughout the years?
- Do you think these titles shape or define your identity?
- What was it like reading the differences between identity and diagnostic language?

LESSON 4: DIAGNOSTIC CRITERIA AND THE IMPACT ON COMMUNITY

Discussion Points

Staying up to date on current research is something that keeps us informed about best practices. The *Diagnostic and Statistical Manual of Mental Disorders V* (*DSM-V*) is the source for experts in the field to utilize for diagnosing people with an array of conditions. Recently, the *DSM-IV* was updated to the *DSM-V* in order to update research and enhance best practices for clinicians. This most recent update completely removed some subtypes of disabilities which left some individuals with a diagnosis of Asperger's feeling uneasy about the shift. One of the most significant changes to ASD in the *DSM-V* is the combining of autism and Asperger's into one category, coded with levels of severity. Although individuals who have been diagnosed under the *DSM-IV* will be able to keep their diagnosis of Asperger's, it creates tension for those that finally were able to connect with a community: the "Aspie" community. In a sense, it appears that some high-functioning students might feel like they are left without a place in the diagnosis. As we discussed in Chapter 2, "by adapting the Identity Criteria in place of Diagnostic Criteria, individuals can hold on to their sense of community." Students will have the opportunity to embrace their strengths and explore the way they can contribute to teams, groups, and in a job.

Guiding Questions

- What are your thoughts about the recent changes in the *DSM-V*?
- What does "Aspie" mean to you?
- What are the negative effects of the changes to the *DSM-V*?
- What are some positives?

LESSON 5: OWNING ASD

Discussion Points

Acceptance is the first step to empowering individuals to be all they can be. Once an individual has accepted that ASD is a part of his or her identity, they begin to shift toward embracing positive qualities, their strengths, and adapting their unique abilities to fit into social norms. They begin to own their ASD. Through the process of owning ASD, individuals can take control and better communicate their needs, which, in return, creates a better life for them and those close to them. The idea is to view ASD in a more positive way while not dismissing some of the challenges faced by individuals on the spectrum. Challenges may always be present, but learning how to advocate is key to overcoming barriers. Some individuals choose to disclose, while some do not. It is important that individuals understand the pros and cons behind disclosing and figure out what works for them. By owning ASD, individuals will begin to better understand themselves, which makes disclosure an easier task when and if disclosing is necessary.

Guiding Questions

- How have you embraced ASD?
- What are some qualities of ASD that you have owned?
- What have been some difficulties in embracing the ASD diagnosis?
- What are some ASD strengths that you can personally connect to?
- Is it difficult for you to disclose to others?
- When might it be important to disclose ASD?
- Has language helped you gain a more positive perspective on ASD?

CHAPTER 3: ASD IN THE MEDIA

LESSON 1: DEVELOPMENT OF PERCEPTIONS THROUGH POPULAR MEDIA

Discussion Points

The media contributes to the way individuals perceive themselves and others. When it comes to ASD, perceptions of this diagnosis are varied and are exhibited through various modes of media. People who have ASD and those who do not have ASD process the messages from the media differently sometimes, and these interpretations impact how ASD is viewed. When students use the messages they receive from the media, it is important that they remember that they are responsible for establishing their perceptions, so distinguishing between positive and negative messages is key to ensuring a positive self-perception of ASD. Processing the impact of the media can be practiced through understanding how neurotypical people are influenced by the media and then considering how these perceptions differ from those of people who have ASD.

Guiding Questions

- How does the media impact perceptions?
- Why is it important to think about how neurotypical people gather information through the media?
- Who can you discuss these perceptions with?
- What are some different media channels that discuss ASD?

LESSON 2: ASD IN THE NEWS

Discussion Points

As young adults, students might be beginning to explore who they are and for what they stand. Our exposure to our environment is considered to be a key factor in understanding the way our surroundings impact us. People gather information from various news sources, each contributing to how they perceive the world around them. Individuals with ASD tend to shape their views with more concrete evidence and are less likely to make judgments based on irrelevant data. One cannot dismiss the fact that others might get their worldviews from media sources, gossip, and various other news sources which might not always include accurate information. Skewed interpretations contribute to negative assumptions within the ASD community. Individuals within the ASD community, whether they are advocates, someone with ASD, or family or friends of someone on the spectrum, might all take active advocacy roles through reactions to new information and judgments passed on the news source. One must recognize their role in making the change as society is starting to shift into projecting a more positive image of ASD. Regardless, media can have long-lasting effects when assumptions are made. Being mindful of how quickly assumptions can be made, educating yourself on the facts before reacting, and being able to determine what makes a source of information reliable is important in navigating some of the misconstrued ideas projected in the media. Students are asked to explore various sources of information and identify misconstrued ideas, false assumptions, or irrelevant details in order to gain a better understanding of how to advocate for ASD.

Guiding Questions

- What are some assumptions you have made about others?
- What are some current events and how does the media portray them?
- What recent news stories have been tied to ASD?
- The media is quick to make assumptions, but hesitates to address mistakes. Can you give an example?
- What are some examples of accurate representation in the media?

LESSON 3: ASD IN MOVIES AND TELEVISION

Discussion Points

Students are asked to reflect on different periods of their life and how they contribute to their self-perceptions. In order to understand how the media portrays individuals with ASD and how this influences self-perceptions, the impact of movies and television shows is discovered in this process. Several famous movies have impacted how ASD is viewed. Characters portray positive characteristics of ASD and some impose false perceptions of an individual with ASD. Script writers work to provide an accurate representation of ASD in occupational and social settings. For students on the spectrum, much can be learned from favorite characters in television shows and movies. In addition to developing an understanding of the genuine qualities of ASD, this also gives a way to normalize their sometimes quirky behavior and understand how things fit into social norms.

Guiding Questions

- In what ways does your personal story relate to Temple Grandin's?
- Like in Temple's experience, mentors can positively impact experiences. Do you currently have someone in your life that understands you and is supportive? Who is it?
- What are some movies that portray a character with ASD?
- Do you relate to Sheldon Cooper from *The Big Bang Theory*? In what ways?
- What are some qualities you share with some of your favorite characters?

LESSON 4: ASD IN SOCIAL MEDIA

Discussion Points

With all the recent advances in technology, we are beginning to see social media replace some of the traditional news sources as the foundation for gathering information on current events. Newspapers and television news sources in society are becoming more obsolete with the increase in social media sharing. Society craves the ability to obtain information immediately and in a more direct manner. The problem lies in whether or not these social media sites are used to provide reliable information. Social media is not monitored or governed, meaning it is often based on someone else's understanding or misconstrued data. Posts to sites can be misinterpreted and cause misunderstandings that easily spread through the internet. Having students discuss how this impacts how others perceive them is important as students learn how to appropriately react. By learning how to advocate through social media sites, students could give society insight to truths and an educated understanding from someone with real ASD knowledge. There is always an appropriate way to advocate, which can be one of the most difficult things to learn, and advocacy is seen as vital in efforts to promote ASD awareness. Students should explore current events and postings that might negatively affect how ASD is understood and think of ways to change that in our society.

Guiding Questions

- What role does social media play in your life?
- How accurate are things you read on social media sites?

- How can you use social media to advocate for yourself?
- What are some examples of negativity you can find on social media sites?
- What are some ways social media can make a difference in your life?
- How can you monitor open communication?

CHAPTER 4: IDENTIFYING YOUR STRENGTHS

LESSON 1: SUCCESS AND ASD QUALITIES

Discussion Points

When students are challenged to recognize their strengths, it can help to see how ASD has influenced the strengths of several successful men and women. Isaac Newton was a rule-follower who kept meticulous work records. Nikola Tesla worked intensely on his interest area and had a few unconventional quirks, like staying in hotel rooms divisible by three. Dan Ackroyd's interest in law enforcement and ghosts contributed to his success in his most famous film role. Daryl Hannah was successful in the movie industry, but was shy and avoided the chaos of her own films' premieres. Taking a look at how these successful individuals with ASD or with ASD characteristics utilized established strengths in ASD is a great first step for students on the spectrum who are working toward understanding their own strengths.

Guiding Questions

- What characteristics of the individuals discussed in the lesson resonate the most with you?
- What strengths do each of these people portray?
- How can you use the strengths of ASD as an individual?
- Do you share any characteristics and strengths with any of the people discussed?

LESSON 2: IDENTIFYING THE ESTABLISHED STRENGTHS IN ASD

Discussion Points

Recognizing strengths can be a difficult task for some students. Students with ASD tend to identify more with their differences by holding on to the negative stigmas they have been exposed to throughout the years. The idea of reframing their negative views about themselves into more positive ones can take time and patience and requires the use of identified strengths. Through the personal stories of students and their various experiences, students have the ability to gain insight into where these stigmas formulated. Now the focus is shifting more toward what makes an individual unique and how those characteristics positively influence the community and those around them. Regardless of what students identify with and what makes them unique, students might find it helps to place emphasis on positive self-perceptions when identifying their strengths.

Guiding Questions

- What established strengths of ASD do you identity with?
- What are some of your strengths?
- How do you project these with confidence?
- What are some things you have learned about your strengths?
- Do you have qualities in common with some famous inventors such as Isaac Newton?

LESSON 3: RECOGNIZING YOUR INDIVIDUAL STRENGTHS

Discussion Points

Individuals with ASD might have a difficult time recognizing some of the behaviors or characteristics generally associated with ASD as strengths. In previous chapters we have talked about the negative impact others can have on how one views oneself. In this section it is more important to identify with those you trust, especially when they are helping to identify positive traits and some areas to improve. Students sometimes view working to identify strengths as a difficult process since it takes time and energy, but once strengths are acknowledged, they can help young adults in all facets of their lives. When an individual understands that there are many ways to think about what makes up individual strengths and how they can be incorporated into their future, intentional decisions and steps can be taken to move forward efficiently. Once an individual with ASD begins to identify their strengths they will begin to explore how these strengths can be utilized at their full potential, contribute to their future career, and influence how they interact with others.

Guiding Questions

- How do your strengths align with your interests?
- How can you gain perspectives through insight?
- How can your strengths contribute to your success?
- In what ways have your strengths contributed to your self-perception?

LESSON 4: REPLACING NEGATIVE SELF-PERCEPTIONS

Discussion Points

Having awareness of and the ability to utilize strengths is essential to the ability to succeed at full potential. If individuals hold on to only negative perceptions, it is likely they will have more negative experiences. Knowing that individuals who have more of a positive outlook are likely to have more positive experiences in their life is an important thing to remember as students approach this time in their lives. Students should spend time exploring what triggers their self-talk and how that contributes to their negative self-perceptions. They must also recognize that there is positive within the negative. Learning how to take the negative self-talk and pull positive things and characteristics from those instances is a common way to gain insight of an individual's strengths. An individual can only do this if they are able to sort out the negative self-talk. After reflecting through the activities the goal should be that students are able to identify their traits and explore the positive benefits of ASD and how those contribute to their day-to-day interactions.

Guding Questions

- What personality traits impact your self-perception?
- What negative self-talk is holding you back?
- What are some things you have learned about your negative self-talk patterns?
- How can you replace these with more positive self-talk?
- In what way can you practice these things?

LESSON 5: REFRAMING YOUR VIEW

Discussion Points

Shifting views can prove to be a daunting task. For students on the spectrum, flexibility of thought can be a common difficulty and might contribute to some frustration with reframing views. Establishing strategies for reframing views is important because maintaining negative attitudes and perspectives on the self or the world is not effective for college students. In order to project confidence in individual strengths and contributions to groups and to work, students with ASD need to let go of any negative views that are encountered. Once strengths have been identified, students can use them as a catalyst through the process of reframing views. Looking at the world through a positive lens allows individuals to recognize and benefit from what they view in the world. Shifting from negative to positive can be difficult, but once it has occurred, students will demonstrate new knowledge of their environment through the positive lens by utilizing the strengths a positive view illustrates for them.

Guiding Questions

- Why is it important to reframe your view to be more positive?
- How can knowing your strengths help with reframing your view?
- How does reframing occur in different settings?
- What is difficult for you about reframing your view?
- Who do you think can help you with this process?

CHAPTER 5: DEVELOPING YOUR CORE IDENTITY

LESSON 1: IDENTIFYING WHAT MAKES YOU CALM, PASSIONATE, AND ANXIOUS

Discussion Points

Core identity can be described as a person's foundation or the building blocks to what makes them who they are at their core. Core values can affect the way one makes decisions, reacts to situations, and even what role one's belief system plays in one's identity. Identifying what makes an individual calm, what drives their passion, and what fuels their anxiety can be a difficult thing to do. In doing so, individuals with ASD can begin to recognize how they present behaviors relating to each topic and how those reactions affect them socially. Students who spend time identifying things that make them calm, passionate, or anxious develop an understanding of what is important to them at their core. The way one reacts to these things is what is most important to adapting to social norms. It is important to recognize that people with ASD can struggle when shifting their views to conform in social situations, but understanding their core values can help as students learn strategies that enable them to do so.

Guiding Questions

- What are some things that calm you down?
- What are the things that you are passionate about?
- What are some things that are important to you but may not be to others?
- How does being calm, passionate, and anxious affect your decision making?
- How do others identify what makes you calm, passionate, and anxious?
- What are some ways you can start to recognize these things in conversation with your peers?

LESSON 2: DEVELOPING YOUR CORE IDENTITY FEATURES

Discussion Points

Now that students have explored their values, the next step is to develop an understanding of how this information can help them identify core features. For most individuals with ASD, there are intense passionate interests. Understanding the values about which one is passionate plays a role in knowing one's core features. It is important to think about these areas and how they impact thoughts, feelings, and actions in day-to-day life. Students must acknowledge how these core values can shift over time, but realize that the overall foundation will stay the same. Taking the time to allow students to identify five values that positively impact who they are serves as a way to produce the fundamental building blocks students can rely on through the college years. Reflecting on one's values might give insight into how the young adult can build a more positive self-perception and more positive interactions with the world around them.

Guiding Questions

- How can your values (discussed in previous chapter) contribute to your core identity?
- In what way are your thoughts, feelings, and actions represented by your core values?
- How can this process help you become a more responsible person?
- What is a value that makes you passionate?
- What might be a personal value that you approach with very little emotional value?
- What are some ways you can begin to self-monitor your behavior?
- How can your identity features contribute to how you act and react?
- What did you identify as your core values?

LESSON 3: IT IS RARELY BLACK AND WHITE

Discussion Points

Individuals with ASD are often considered black-and-white thinkers. Students tend to think in absolute styles and struggle with flexibility. As students begin to embrace the college experience, they will soon figure out that very few things are actually black and white. It is important to encourage students to explore their core identity features because they will be challenged by having to develop flexibility of thought and view things in a more abstract manner. By using the gray scale visual, students learn and begin to understand how others make decisions and recognize that addressing everything they disagree with is not the way to develop and foster healthy relationships.

Guiding Questions

- What are some examples of an absolute style of thinking?
- How can rigid thinking negatively impact your college experience?
- What are some examples of how you can become more flexible in your thoughts?
- Consider one of your identified core values. How can this impact your decision making?
- How can black-and-white thinking impact your relationships?

LESSON 4: THE INTERSECTION OF YOUR CORE IDENTITY FEATURES

Discussion Points

While exploring how one's values are adhered to by an individual with rigid thinking, the idea of intersecting these core identify features is introduced. The use of realistic scenarios in the chapter demonstrates how intersection of core identity features occurs. Understanding that there is a way for two values to intersect is important. Acknowledging whether or not individuals can project each in a manageable way is something that takes time and commitment to develop. By remaining in a rigid way of thinking, one can see this process as confusing and uncomfortable. The purpose of acknowledging the intersection of core identity features is to challenge students to become more flexible, while remaining true to their values and core identity.

Guiding Questions

- How can core values intersect with each other?
- What are some things you could do to recognize some current black-and-white thinking?
- What is an example of when your values have intersected?
- How can you have flexible thoughts but still stay true to your core?

CHAPTER 6: SOCIAL RULES AND SOCIAL CONFUSION

LESSON 1: SOCIAL CONFUSION AND ESTABLISHING PURPOSE

Discussion Points

Gathering information within the social context of one's life and developing social strategies can be difficult for individuals on the autism spectrum. From this point forward students must understand that the increase of social interactions and evolving transitions will bring up situations that involve social confusion. Young adults must learn how to navigate through these experiences in order to be successful and maintain healthy relationships whether they are career-based or personal. Students must remember that social rules are cultural constructs not universal truths meaning they will shift throughout the course of one's life and experiences. Social rules shift from situation to situation, but, with the use of the five tools discussed in the chapter, students can learn how to utilize social strategies affectively. Exploring social miscues, initial reactions, solutions, and ways to recharge will help an individual process through a situation of social confusion. How to navigate through these steps will influence their development of social miscue awareness.

Guiding Questions

- What have you learned about social norms on a college campus?
- What are some social rules that you can identify and how do you adhere to those in social situations?
- What might be a good example of social confusion?
- Why do you think understanding social rules will be beneficial to your career?
- Can you identify a time when you found yourself really confused about how to react to something social?
- What does it mean to have social awareness?
- What does it mean for relationships to be dynamic? Can you give an example of this?
- How could you identify a social miscue?

LESSON 2: RULES OF SOCIAL ENGAGEMENT

Discussion Points

Individuals with ASD often experience social confusion which keeps them from interacting with peers, especially on a college campus. For neurotypicals, it seems a relatively easy task to navigate through the social world around them. For individuals with ASD, unpredictable social interaction can prove to be more of a difficult process and this often serves as the reasoning behind students failing to engage in much social interaction at all. By exploring the Rules of Social Engagement, one might realize that social interactions can have a positive impact. Although rules are not absolute factors, they will serve as guidelines for engaging socially while also conforming to social expectations. Recognizing simple rules including "first impressions are vital," "manners matter," "people adapt to situations," "everyone serves a purpose," and "relationships are dynamic," students will have a baseline in how to socially engage.

Guiding Questions

- What are some social challenges you have faced?
- How can you use the social rules to help you navigate through social interactions?
- What impressions do you have of those around you?
- What impressions do you think you leave with others?
- What can you do to navigate through some of the social confusion in your life?
- What manners do you utilize daily to help you fit in socially?
- How might interacting with a friend be different from interacting with a professor?
- Give an example of why you would socially shift in a situation with your peers.
- What is something significant you have to offer to your peers? What is something they could have to offer you?

LESSON 3: BUILDING YOUR SOCIAL FIRST AID KIT

Discussion Points

A first aid kit serves to help when situations are minor and can be utilized when treating small scrapes or mild bruises, but can also be the initial resource in a serious emergency until medical help is obtained. The same idea holds true for a social first aid kit. If you have the tools you need there when you need them, they may help in the case of an emergency. It is helpful if students on the spectrum have detailed descriptions or examples to follow when navigating new experiences. Students use tools to explore the idea of utilizing their resources. In this case, tools are designed to quickly help young adults navigate through common social situations. In the kit, tools such as social consultants, social study guides, skills mapping, scripts, and social dissection can be used in various situations and have long-lasting impacts on how individuals engage socially. In times of crisis one might not be able to process information quickly and effectively. The emergency manual is there to give students a sense of direction when emergency strikes. Each tool plays an important part in helping students on the spectrum better understand the steps in navigating the social world.

Guiding Questions

- What are some tools that you could use to help you navigate through a social miscue that might happen in a classroom setting?
- What has your reaction been during a time where you were experiencing social confusion?

- Who could you identify as a social consultant?
- What do you keep in your social first aid kit in addition to the tools mentioned in the chapter?
- What is a social miscue that can happen for individuals with ASD?
- What are some ways you could resolve a social misunderstanding?
- How can you create your own social study guide?
- Think of something that happened to you today and perform a social dissection.
- What plans can you make for emergency situations?

LESSON 4: DIGGING YOUR WAY OUT

Discussion Points

Even though students have access to tools and resources, they can still end up stuck as a result of a social miscue. Their ability to find their way out of bad situations is something that will be beneficial to their future success as roadblocks are inevitable. A social hole could be the result of a social miscue. Students must start by setting their emotions aside and following a few simple steps in order to learn from their experience and move past it. When stuck in a social hole, students must take the time to acknowledge what has happened and how it has impacted those around them. They must then engage in effective communication to assess the damage that was caused and what response is needed. Student must then use tools presented throughout this chapter to respond to the situation and determine how they plan to effectively work toward digging their way out. It is vital that students understand that if they do not see results they must try a different approach. After identifying the best response they must re-evaluate the damage done, try to repair it, but most importantly move on. These five steps help someone with ASD work their way out of various situations in which they feel stuck and help repair the damage caused. This section combines all of Chapter 4 into a simple five-step approach that if utilized correctly can dig students out.

Guiding Questions

- Can you identify a time when you have felt stuck in a social hole?
- How do you resolve a social miscue? What are the steps?
- How can you implement strategies from this chapter?
- How will you use these strategies to reach the potential you have in your career?

CHAPTER 7: BUILDING YOUR TEAM

LESSON 1: UNDERSTANDING YOUR PREFERENCES

Discussion Points

For some individuals with ASD, there can be many challenges when working with a team which can occur not only in the college setting, but also in one's career. Individuals with ASD tend to steer clear of teamwork because it can be seen as stressful and not worth the time and effort. As students navigate college and life after, they must understand that working in a team setting is inevitable. One way to make the process of working with a team easier is to understand preferences when it comes to others and how they contribute. Knowing oneself and how best to work in a team setting would create less conflict and be seen as less taxing on your energy. It is important for students to remember lessons learned up to this point and how those lessons play a part in the process of acknowledging what works best for an individual.

Guiding Questions

- What do you look for when establishing a team?
- Looking over the activity, where do you fall on the spectrum for each category?
- Can you think of the benefits to having several different personalities/styles on a team?
- In your opinion, how does a group best operate?
- How flexible are you in group activities?
- What could be identified as a weakness?

LESSON 2: RECOGNIZING THE PREFERENCES OF OTHERS

Discussion Points

Part 1 of the process is identifying an individual's preferences and how they contribute to a team. The next step is encouraging students to explore the preferences of others and discuss why this knowledge is important. A key thing to remember is "there is no I in team," and while the saying may be a cliché, it is a good reminder for those students who are focused on themselves more than their team members. The goal is to determine what makes a successful team, what the other person contributes, and what works well with the needs of someone on the spectrum.

Guiding Questions

- Do you get anxious when you know you have to work in a team?
- What different perspectives can you contribute?

- What preferences make a good match for you?
- How can you approach someone you know you would work well with?

LESSON 3: PARTNERING PREFERENCES TO BUILD TEAMS

Discussion Points

The goal when partnering preferences to build teams is to determine the needs of the individual as well as the needs of the other team members. Through analyzing the strengths and preferences of both an individual and others in a group, students can help structure an effective group setting. This allows students to reflect on past experiences to better optimize future group involvement. It is important to explore the notion that good teams do not only consist of members with the same skill set and experiences. Teamwork, whether in an academic setting or a career setting, will always have potential pitfalls. By having awareness and knowledge of the preferences of team members, individuals are more likely to have a positive impact on a team.

Guiding Questions

- Do you think you contribute your unique input when working in teams?
- Can you name a time when you have had to collaborate with someone outside of schoolwork?
- How easy is it for you to communicate with others on your team?
- What does a good partnership look like to you?

LESSON 4: ROLES IN WORK TEAMS/GROUPS

Discussion Points

Often students with ASD fail to realize the benefits of being on a team. Up to this point students have been challenged to explore their preferences and what best works for them in a team setting. Now students are being asked to define specific roles and benefits of teamwork. There are benefits to being the motivator, the analyzer, the harmonizer and the taskmaster but having each group member identify with a role is key to having successful groups. By addressing the preferences of others and how these are reflected in the roles described in the chapter, students can work for a more cohesive group experience using what was learned for future group involvement.

Guiding Questions

- What is challenging to you when working as a team?
- When thinking of the four roles, what stands out most to you?

- If you are not a motivator, how can you find motivation?
- When working on a team, how important is harmony?
- How does a taskmaster positively contribute to a team?
- What are you looking for in a team?
- What working style best fits your needs?
- What kind of environment is conducive to your style?
- How can you communicate these things to others effectively?

CHAPTER 8: CHANGING THE GOAL

LESSON 1: LOOKING FORWARD

Discussion Points

Before students can take steps toward a career, they need to figure out where they stand in terms of academic logistics, like grade point average and credit hours required for graduation. These are daunting steps for some students who do like to think too far into the future, but tending to these tasks allows for a much easier shift to career preparation. Leaning on the support of academic advisors, disability services, career planning services, and mentors, students can adjust any logistical need they might have and move to the next step. For many students, the early part of college is a time of transition and new experiences. As students settle in, though, it is easy to become complacent in terms of planning for the next few years. Proactive measures can be taken to improve the process of preparing for a career, as this process typically occurs simultaneously with increased academic demands. Students must realize that as they progress through their academic career, the demands for their higher level courses will impact how they spend their time and energy. Adding in the element of career preparation can make this feel overwhelming. Looking forward and taking care of academic logistics as a college student will ensure that students are prepared to spend more time investing in community services, internships, and job shadowing, which will ultimately increase their marketability for future employment.

Guiding Questions

- What are some concrete steps that you can take to prepare for a career?
- What do we mean when we say "logistics for your career"?
- Do you have a current résumé?
- What can you add to your résumé to update it?
- Describe something that you've discovered about yourself that makes you marketable.

- Who can you identify as a person to lean on through this process?
- What kind of support do you have? What does that support look like?
- Have you thought about what potential employers will expect you to have when you graduate (GPA, experience)?
- What are realistic goals you want to set for yourself?
- What benefits from some of your general education courses can you identify as good experience?

LESSON 2: CHOOSING THE RIGHT ACADEMIC MAJOR

Discussion Points

The academic major guides coursework through college. Choosing a major that is both interesting academically and practical for you and your career goals is an essential step for young adults in college. Students can use what they know about their strengths, values, and interests to pursue a meaningful academic courseload. For some, making the commitment to a specific academic focus can be difficult. For others, it will ensure that interest levels remain high throughout their time at college. There are many elements to this decision, though, and it should not simply be made from a face-value point of view. Many interesting academic programs are designed differently on different campuses. For example, one academic program may be practical and lab based, while another is centered on discussion. Learning about your potential options allows students to make a decision that fits their needs and interests more holistically.

Guiding Questions

- How can your special interest contribute to your academic major choice?
- What motivates your academic success?
- How does this motivation contribute outside of the classroom?
- In what way does your knowledge go beyond academics?
- What can you identify as your purpose and main focus?
- Is committing to the future difficult for you?
- What can you identify as some interest-driven social interactions at your college?

LESSON 3: THE CAREER CONTINUUM

Discussion Points

The Career Continuum in Chapter 8 is a progression of common and proven career preparation elements. While these four elements—community service, supervised internship, major internship, and career—are not always present in students' plans for career preparation, having a basic understanding of their potential benefit for career-focused students allows for opportunities to seek career experience while in college. First, students will learn about community service and its value in the career preparation process. Then students will develop an understanding of the difference between a supervised internship and a major internship and what the potential benefits are of each. Lastly, students will explore what "career" actually means. Knowing what each of these steps are helps students to choose which proven elements can be goals for them as they move through their academic coursework.

Guiding Questions

- How can you plan to build your experience outside of the classroom?
- Do you have any experience with community service?
- What are some ways you can continue or start building your community service experience?
- What is the benefit of community services engagements?
- How can you begin to plan for the idea of supervised internships?
- What would be the benefit of doing so?
- Can you think of possible internship sites that you would be interested in?
- When thinking about workplace environment, what can you identify as being important?
- How could that change or be adapted?
- What is the difference between supervised internships and major internships?
- How can your role as an intern help prompt you to a successful career?
- How do you define "career"?
- How can previous experience be of assistance to your future career?
- In what way can you begin to create your own path?
- How can you adapt this Career Continuum idea to your situation and long- and short-term goals?

LESSON 4: AN INTRODUCTION TO COMMUNITY SERVICE, JOB SHADOWING, AND INTERNSHIPS

Discussion Points

Taking the time to explore potential opportunities that can help prepare students for a career is worthwhile as it exposes the possible options for relevant experience necessary for a career. In this introduction to community service, job shadowing, and internships, students work through any previous experience they have that has opened doors for new opportunities in their chosen field. There are differing levels of responsibility and engagement required in each of the three career preparation possibilities discussed in this chapter. Building experience through any one or all three of these possibilities will positively impact students' résumés and overall career readiness. The experience provides students with invaluable insight into the field or fields they are interested in. For these opportunities, students will probably have to interview and apply for the chance to learn in their field. While this might seem daunting, it is practice for the interviews students will encounter in their job search. These opportunities also allow students who are choosing between a few academic majors to explore potential fields connected with their major. In a sense, community service, job shadowing, and internship opportunities can be looked at as interviews for potential fields.

Guiding Questions

- What is meant by "career relevant experience"?
- In what ways have you started building the experience you need?
- If you have not started or have limited previous experience, what can you do to change that?
- How would job shadowing be a good experience?
- What are the differences in the "three common stepping stones" (page 180) mentioned in the chapter?
- What kind of deadlines can you expect during the process?

LESSON 5: MENTORS AND CAREER PREPARATION

Discussion Points

Understanding the role of a professional mentor and how a mentor can help students with career preparation is the focus of this lesson. Since students have worked through social strategies geared toward intentional interactions, the mentor can be a safe outlet for students to practice these strategies. Knowing how to choose a mentor is also important as students will want to have a good and effective match. Once a mentorship has been established, students must work with their mentor to develop guidelines for their interactions, such as how frequently the pair will meet and what the focus of the interactions will be. These guidelines will allow the student to ensure they have the input of their mentor in all career aspects about which they need feedback. In terms of career preparation, students with ASD will need to build their resume throughout their college experience and also make a point to practice interviewing. These two career preparation pieces will be imperative as students embark on the job search and application process, which will probably take place in the last few semesters of college, if not before then. Taking advantage of the help a mentor can provide is something that all college students would benefit from, but students with ASD will also gain social feedback and practice in a structured partnership, making each step of the process more approachable.

Guiding Questions

- Do you have a professional mentor?
- If not, how do you identify people that you could lean on for support?
- What can your professional mentor contribute to your career preparation?
- What boundaries or guidelines should you establish, or have you established, with your professional mentor?
- What are your expectations in a mentorship?
- How can you anticipate making time in your schedule for a mentor?
- What are some characteristics in a mentor that would be good for you?

REFERENCES

American Psychiatric Association (2013) *Diagnostic and Statistical Manual of Mental Disorders (Fifth Edition)*. Washington, DC: American Psychiatric Association.

Attwood, T. (1998) *Asperger's Syndrome: A Guide for Parents and Professionals.* London: Jessica Kingsley Publishers.

Attwood T. (1999). The Discovery of "Aspie" Criteria. www.tonyattwood.com.au/index.php?option=com_content&view=article&id=79%3Athe-discovery-of-aspie-criteria, accessed on 3 March 2015.

Chiang, H.-M., Cheung, K., Hickson, L., Xiang, R. and Tsai, L. (2012). Predictive factors of participation in postsecondary education for high school leavers with autism. *Journal of Autism and Developmental Disorders 42,* 685–696.

Cooper, G. F. (2013) "Daryl Hannah: I've battled autism since childhood." Available at www.today.com/popculture/daryl-hannah-ive-battled-autism-childhood-8C11278435, accessed on 5 January 2015.

Fitzgerald, M. and O'Brien, B. (2007) *Genius Genes.* Shawnee Mission, KS: Autism Asperger Publishing Company.

Grandin, T. (2011) *The Way I See It: A Personal Look at Autism and Asperger's.* Arlington, TX: Future Horizons, Inc.

Grandin, T. and Barron, S. (2005) *The Unwritten Rules of Social Relationships: Decoding Social Mysteries Through the Unique Perspectives of Autism.* Arlington, TX: Future Horizons, Inc.

Iles, G. (1906) *Inventors at Work.* New York, NY: Doubleday, Page.

Marcia, J. E. (2002) Identity and psychosocial development in adulthood. *Identity: An International Journal of Theory and Research 2,* 1, 7–28.

Miller, C. (2013) Dan Aykroyd says being on the spectrum helped him make Ghostbusters. Available at www.childmind.org/en/press/brainstorm/dan-aykroyd-credits-autism-helping-him-make-ghostb, accessed on 5 January 2015.

Roybal, J. (2008). Temple Grandin talks about her upcoming HBO biopic. http://beefmagazine.com/cowcalfweekly/1031-temple-grandin-hbo-biopic, accessed on 3 March 2015.

Wallis, C. (2010). Temple Grandin on Temple Grandin. http://content.time.com/time/arts/article/0,8599,1960347,00.html, accessed on 3 March 2015.

Wolf, L. E., Brown, J. T. and Bork, G. R. K. (2009) *Students with Asperger Syndrome: A Guide for College Personnel.* Shawnee Mission, KS: Autism Asperger Publishing Company.

INDEX

Made in the USA
Lexington, KY
20 April 2016